T0183654

Health Behavior Change in the Dental Practice

HEALTH BEHAVIOR CHANGE IN THE DENTAL PRACTICE

Edited by
Christoph A. Ramseier and Jean E. Suvan

WILEY-BLACKWELL

A John Wiley & Sons, Inc., Publication

Edition first published 2010
© 2010 Christoph A. Ramseier

Blackwell Publishing was acquired by John Wiley & Sons in February 2007. Blackwell's
publishing program has been merged with Wiley's global Scientific, Technical, and Medical
business to form Wiley-Blackwell.

Editorial Office
2121 State Avenue, Ames, Iowa 50014-8300, USA

For details of our global editorial offices, for customer services, and for information about
how to apply for permission to reuse the copyright material in this book, please see our
Website at www.wiley.com/wiley-blackwell.

Authorization to photocopy items for internal or personal use, or the internal or personal use
of specific clients, is granted by Blackwell Publishing, provided that the base fee is paid directly
to the Copyright Clearance Center, 222 Rosewood Drive, Danvers, MA 01923. For those
organizations that have been granted a photocopy license by CCC, a separate system of
payments has been arranged. The fee code for users of the Transactional Reporting Service is
ISBN-13: 978-0-8138-2106-1/2010.

Library of Congress Cataloging-in-Publication Data

Health behavior change in the dental practice / editors, Christoph A. Ramseier and
Jean E. Suvan.
p. ; cm.
Includes bibliographical references and index.
ISBN 978-0-8138-2106-1 (pbk. : alk. paper)
1. Dental health education. 2. Health behavior. 3. Behavior modification. 4. Dental
personnel and patient. I. Ramseier, Christoph A. II. Suvan, Jean E.
[DNLM: 1. Oral Health. 2. Health Behavior. 3. Health Education–
methods. 4. Motivation. 5. Professional-Patient Relations. WU 113 H4339 2010]
RK60.8.H43 2010
617.6071–dc22
2010013920

A catalog record for this book is available from the U.S. Library of Congress.

Set in 10 on 12.5pt Sabon by Toppan Best-set Premedia Limited

1   2010

To my precious son, AJ, and my dear husband, Bob
For your endless unconditional love and support, for giving so much
meaning to my life.
J.E.S.

To my late grandmother, Hedwig
For the ongoing inspiration you have given me to pursue academia.

To my parents, Rosmarie and Ernst, my sister, Andrea, and her children,
Michèle and Joel
In appreciation of your unwavering love.
Ch.A.R.

CONTENTS

There's a very common challenge that we all face, at work and at home, when it comes to encouraging behavior change in other people: we might want them to do this or that, we might encourage, request, ask, implore, beg, or instruct, but in the end, only they can change their behavior; we can't do it for them. Then there's our own behavior change, and the struggles we all know about when we try to change ourselves. What has helped us? If we were a patient, what would we find useful and not so helpful?

These questions arise every day in dental practice, and you will recognize the common patterns in the reports of practitioners across the board:

"I just wish he would look after his gums better".

"If only he could see what I can see. There's trouble coming."

"If he doesn't do his side of the bargain, it's tough for me to do mine."

"Smoking: well, it's just a problem, and I don't know how many times I have told them that it's a good plan to quit."

The problem is, people don't just change their behavior because someone else gives them information that this will be a good idea. You can't instill motivation to change into someone else!

One of the challenges we must face is that motivation to change is not a black-white phenomenon, but something that comes in degrees, with most people feeling ambivalent about change. They can see reasons to change and they can also see reasons not to change. This makes them quite sensitive to how they are spoken to, and this is where something like Motivational Interviewing can be of help. If you try to persuade people who are feeling ambivalent that they might, should, or could change, their natural inclination is to give voice to the counterargument, why they can't change. This "resistant" reaction is not just their fault; it's partly to do with how you approach the conversation. Put bluntly, it's better if they, rather than you, say why and how they could change.

This book is the first of its kind to take these observations and ideas into the world of everyday dental practice. It's full of useful suggestions and things to try out, and most important, it's a resource book for students and practitioners in every field of dental care. Learn how to handle these sometimes tricky conversations about behavior change, and your consultations will feel less frustrating and much more rewarding. Evidence about effectiveness is emerging, and this book could also provide the inspiration for researchers in the years to come.

I wish the authors and particularly those practitioners out there good luck and happier consultations.

Stephen Rollnick
Professor of Health Care Communication
Department of Primary Care and Public Health
Cardiff University, Wales, UK

PREFACE

Following the publication of the chapter on Motivational Interviewing in the fifth edition of Jan Lindhe's textbook on *Clinical Periodontology and Implant Dentistry*, we felt highly inspired to expand the topic of health behavior change within the dental profession. In agreement with the publisher, a new book was to be written specifically designed for dental clinicians as a tool to enable and facilitate the implementation of health behavior change counselling in their everyday patient care.

In order to meet this goal, a multi-disciplinary team of co-authors was carefully selected. We are proud that our book reflects a unique collaboration between dental clinicians and health behavior change psychologists. Countless meetings, phone calls, and e-mails between the co-authors, over the past 3 years, have enabled the creation of the work presented here. Compared to common textbooks in the dental field, the content of this book presents and elaborates a different philosophy of patient care for clinicians. While the book focuses on patient behavior change, it carries the potential to change the dental professional as well—for example, by changing the clinicians' approach from "asking closed questions" to "asking open questions" or from "giving instructions to the patient" to "actively listening to the patient's needs."

The reader will notice that most chapters have been created and edited as a team effort. As a result of this close collaboration and exchange amongst all the authors, we have been able to formulate and present a concept of health behavior change counselling compatible with the dental setting.

As we reflect on the journey taken to prepare this book, the influence and time invested by our many colleagues and mentors, too numerous to name, who have played a role in our development as dental professionals is greatly appreciated. There is one person, Klaus Lang, who cannot remain unnamed due to the unparalleled impact he has had on each of us as a committed guide in our professional careers.

We would also like to specifically acknowledge the support of Steve Rollnick, who always made himself available for thought-provoking discussions. We are deeply grateful to Bob Suvan and Angela Fundak for providing candid criticism and insightful suggestions based on their diligent proofreading of numerous drafts. In addition, we express our sincere appreciation to our families for their unending support and encouragement.

Finally, we would like to express our gratitude to Sophia Joyce from Wiley-Blackwell for her constructive assistance and patience in allowing us the time necessary to complete this endeavor.

Christoph A. Ramseier

Jean E. Suvan

Vanessa Bogle, DPsych, MSc, BSc
Health Psychologist
Department of Psychology
City University
Northampton Square
London
EC1V 0HB
United Kingdom

Delwyn Catley, PhD
Professor
Department of Psychology
University of Missouri–Kansas City
5100 Rockhill Road
Kansas City, MO 64110-2499

Angela Fundak, RDH, GDAET
Sorella Communications
PO Box 187
Prahran 3181, Victoria
Australia

Nina Gobat, BA, BSc
Department of Primary Care and
  Public Health
School of Medicine
Cardiff University
7th Floor Neuadd Meirionnydd
Heath Park
Cardiff
CF14 4YS
United Kingdom

Kathy Goggin, PhD
Professor
Department of Psychology
University of Missouri–Kansas City
5100 Rockhill Road
Kansas City, MO 64110-2499

Anne Koerber, DDS, PhD
Associate Professor
University of Illinois at Chicago
College of Dentistry, Pediatric
  Dentistry
801 S. Paulina, MC 850
Chicago, IL 60612

Claire Lane, PhD
Trainee Clinical Psychologist
University of Birmingham
School of Psychology
Edgbaston
Birmingham
B15 2TT
United Kingdom

Ian Lynam, PhD
Department of Psychology
University of Missouri–Kansas
  City
5100 Rockhill Road
Kansas City, MO 64110-2499

Christoph A. Ramseier, Dr. med.
  dent., MAS
Assistant Professor
University of Berne
School of Dental Medicine
Department of Periodontology
Freiburgstrasse 7
CH-3010 Bern
Switzerland

Philip S. Richards, DDS, MS
Clinical Professor
Division of Periodontology
Department of Periodontics and
  Oral Medicine
University of Michigan School of
  Dentistry
1101 N. University Avenue
Ann Arbor, MI 48109-1078

Jean E. Suvan, DipDH, MSc, CRA,
  FHEA
Clinical Research Coordinator
Periodontology Unit
Division of Restorative Dental
  Services
UCL Eastman Dental Institute
256 Gray's Inn Road
London WC1X 8LD
United Kingdom

Health Behavior Change in the Dental Practice

CHAPTER 1

INTRODUCTION TO HEALTH BEHAVIOR CHANGE FOR THE DENTAL PRACTICE

Christoph A. Ramseier, Jean Suvan, Angela Fundak, and Philip S. Richards

HEALTH CARE IN THE TWENTY-FIRST CENTURY

Health professionals working in this century are presented with a unique combination of patient care scenarios. The unprecedented advances in the development of scientific knowledge, means of knowledge dissemination, clinical skills application, public health initiatives, and workforce diversity are well recognized in today's health care environment. However, many additional factors influence the opportunity for patients and clinicians alike to achieve the goal of attaining health and continued wellness. Some of these may be derived from catastrophic events associated with the conflicts of war, natural disasters, and critical socio-economic factors. Others are more reflective of circumstances for individuals and the lifestyle choices they make throughout their lifetime. In many situations, health status is not a result of the influence of a single element working in isolation. It is more likely that we see a number of components present in the overall environment in which the patient chooses to exist. The acknowledgement of the potential impact of a variety of influences on health status allows the health professional to work with the patient to understand the individual approach for optimal wellness. As oral health professionals, this recognition is integral to the future development of patient care plans that are not limited to treating the signs and symptoms of common dental diseases.

There is increasing evidence suggesting oral health status can affect general health and quality of life in people of all ages. Most oral diseases are common chronic diseases and are momentous public health issues with a high prevalence across all populations worldwide. Some of the etiologies of oral diseases are well known. They include (1) the causal factors induced by oral biofilms, and (2) the lifestyle risk factors common to a number of chronic diseases: insufficient oral hygiene, tobacco use, diet, behaviors causing injuries, and stress. All of these elements are modifiable and associated with the influence of health behaviors as determinants of disease prevalence.

As we are living in a century of heightened awareness of chronic diseases, health care challenges are becoming more diverse, with an increasing percentage of the population in the developed world being diagnosed with health decline associated with "lifestyle" behaviors. Therefore, the health professional is continuously presented with a dual focus—control of current disease while facilitating the understanding of continuous self-management as part of an effective and equitable long-term solution. Oral health professionals are not exempt from this approach to patient care as we continue our efforts to manage common oral diseases as a chronic condition rather than simply

INTRODUCTION

treating the sequelae of acute episodes. This introductory chapter sets the stage for this book through a discussion of past, current, and future understanding of the dental clinician as a health professional supporting the promotion of total health rather than a provider of operative dentistry alone.

There is substantial evidence that oral health can be maintained by adequate behaviors such as regular oral hygiene, avoidance of tobacco, and consumption of a healthy diet. Future public health policies should be reoriented to incorporate oral health practices recommending behavioral support and the common risk factor approach for health promotion. Oral health care professionals should gain an understanding of the health effects of inappropriate behaviors in order to successfully target prevention and disease control. As a consequence, services for primary and secondary prevention on an individual level oriented toward the change of inappropriate behavior will become a professional responsibility for all oral health care providers.

From a practical point of view, it may be preferable to apply methods for health behavior change counselling in oral care that are shown to be effective in both primary and secondary prevention of oral diseases. These methods should be

• based on the best available evidence,

• applicable to oral hygiene behavior, tobacco use prevention and cessation, and dietary counselling, and

• suitable for implementation by the dental practice team in a cost-effective way.

THE OPPORTUNITY IN THE DENTAL SETTING

The dental setting provides a unique environment for the provision of care for a range of health issues. For some time, in many developed nations, people have tended to visit the dental practice more frequently than they visit the medical practitioner. They have been more likely to seek medical advice when they are experiencing discomfort or have recognized symptoms that require assistance. The concept of the regular, 6-month "dental check-up" has enjoyed strong recognition and relevance with many members of the public. In more recent times, health practitioners and public health care initiatives have embraced the concept of regular visits as part of a monitoring/preventive approach rather than a response to an acute episode. This frequency of visitation has allowed collaborative patient care plans to develop with interprofessional exchange. For example, many optometrists regularly screen for signs of diabetic retinopathy as a possible indicator of undiagnosed diabetes or as a consequence of managed diabetes. Within the context of the dental setting, a patient may be a part of the practice for many years and, in some cases, a lifetime. Additionally, the practice may also provide care for the patient's family members and their friends, who all form part of the individual's environment and lifestyle. This unique situation allows the oral health professional to acknowledge and gain a broad understanding of the myriad of influential health care factors associated with patient care. The dental setting, therefore, provides a privileged situation in which the dental professional can realize the opportunity to form a long-standing and supportive relationship in health care management with his or her patient. However, this opportunity is often under-utilized or ignored completely when the clinician assumes a more conventional role.

Historically, dental clinicians have been characterized as "active," "powerful," and "expert," while patients have been described as "passive" and "cooperative." The dental treatment room itself, where the patients are in a submissive position and the clinicians are in a controlling position, supports these traditional roles. With a focus on technical expertise, dental clinicians may believe that their communications with patients will be based on common sense or are secondary to the provision of successful treatment. As shown in Figure 1.1, this traditional view of dental care is generally understood as operative oral medicine, or even dental surgery alone. Even though a patient suffering from oral pain will be correctly diagnosed with a hopeless tooth by the clinician, and subsequently treated with a tooth extraction, the patient may not be approached any further with the measures necessary for the prevention of further tooth loss.

Even if the need for preventive measures is recognized, some dental clinicians struggle with interviewing skills, may miscalculate how much (and how) information should be shared, have difficulty detecting and resolving issues with patient cooperation, or have varying levels of skill in interpreting non-verbal behaviors. Quite possibly due to a familiarity with diagnosing a problem, followed by providing a solution, preventive approaches are delivered in a prescriptive format. This may result in a situation that is illustrated in Figure 1.2: tobacco use is identified in the health history form of a patient who will be approached with the advice to quit. However, since there are no further measures taken, doubt remains whether beneficial health behavior change, such as smoking cessation, will occur.

INTRODUCTION

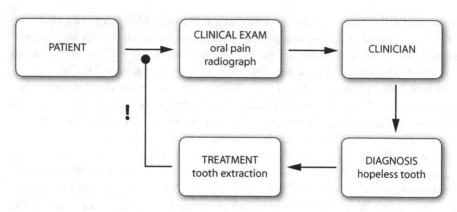

Figure 1.1. Operative oral medicine.

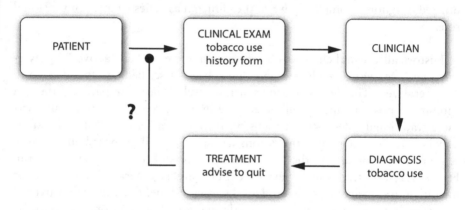

Figure 1.2. Preventive oral medicine.

Consequently, current advice-giving or health education approaches appear to be unpredictable in accomplishing long-term change, potentially leading to frustration of both the patient and the clinician. Yet, the patient may be blamed for poor compliance and further oral health education may be judged as pointless.

Adoption and integration of health behavior change

History has demonstrated that the past efforts of health professionals to promote changes in behavior that support positive health outcomes have potential for improvement. Compliance with medical recommendations is generally poor across all chronic disease regimens, which increases health care expenditures and prevents patients from achieving the full benefit of health behavior interventions. A number of studies have been conducted investigating ways to improve compliance, but research results have not shown to affect significant changes in compliance behavior (Berg et al. 2006).

This dilemma of patient and clinician agreement regarding long-term changes in health behavior has been systematically examined for over 50 years. In 2001, the World Health Organization (WHO) convened a conference to focus on the issues associated with outcomes commonly termed as treatment adherence and compliance. Poor adherence to treatment of chronic diseases was reported at a rate of 50% in developed countries with even lower rates of adherence in developing countries (WHO 2003). This review not only demonstrates the challenges associated with health behavior change but also provides a catalyst for health practitioners to review their role as a significant factor in the success of compliance strategies.

Health care providers may harbor an unwarranted sense of their own importance in inspiring behavior change, ignoring other variables that impact a patient's behavior. This may serve to diminish the patients' key role rather than empowering the patients themselves. Although health care professionals typically believe that they are providing quality care, it is generally from their own perspective that they are defining quality (Larsen et al. 2006). The patient perspective of quality could be very different, as there may be a fundamental disagreement of needs and expectations in the clinician-patient relationship. Even if there is agreement, the acceptance of care or behavior change (adoption) and the practical application (integration) of care or behavior change often requires further exploration to ensure ongoing success.

Many oral health professionals underestimate the importance of communication as compared to technical skill. This tends to foster a focus on compliance rather than collaboration. Additionally, the framework of dental care delivery reinforces a traditional model of clinician-patient roles that diminishes the value of the communication necessary for successful partnership (Gochman 1997). Despite the possible negativity associated with past approaches, oral health professionals should be encouraged, knowing they operate in an environment that is extremely conducive to success. The nature, frequency, and longevity of clinician-patient interaction within the dental setting are unlike any other health care environment. Therefore, the opportunity to work with patients toward the adoption and integration of positive health behaviors into their current lifestyle is limitless. As oral health

INTRODUCTION

professionals choose to take advantage of this privileged situation, they will find themselves valuable providers of integral support across the complete spectrum of health care.

The role and responsibility of the dental professional

Ethical

The ethical basis of interactions with patients to guide behavioral change still needs to be defined. Health care delivery requires competent clinical practice by professionals and avoidance of negative responses by patients that such interventions may induce (such as confusion or loss of self-confidence).

Health behavior change interventions must be devoid of gender, ethnic, cultural, and age bias and designed to be effective for persons of widely varied levels of formal education (Redman 2007). The patient must be an active participant and must willingly engage in the change process. Health care professionals who impose their own values and beliefs on the patient limit the patient's possibilities and create situations of domination and dependence. Ultimately the patient has the ethical right to choose whether or not to change, to choose when to change, and to determine what form any change will take (Chin 2006).

Legal

The legal basis of all interactions with patients directed at guiding behavioral change has been established through case law, regulations governing professional practice, and prescribed requirements for health care institutions. It is particularly guided by the doctrine of informed decision making and consent (Redman 2007).

In the United States, the Joint Commission on the Accreditation of Healthcare Organizations (JCAHO) and the Centers for Medicare & Medicaid Services (CMS) mandate both patient and family education for hospitals and long-term care facilities that are participating in CMS programs. These mandates include the need for documentation of patient education during hospitalization. The organizational structure of such hospitals provides an infrastructure by which coordination, counselling, and documentation may occur for the institution to meet the JCAHO standards

(Rankin et al. 2005). In order for smaller health care organizations (including dental clinics) to meet these goals, the leadership must demonstrate its need. To date, in the United States, no policies or educational guidelines exist for dental care provided outside of hospital settings. Changes in dental professionals' behavior, in education or practice, typically have been slow unless they are regulated or have a potential impact on livelihood (Gift and White 1997).

Collaborative care toward whole health

Historically, the dental profession has suffered as a result of its isolation from others working in health-related fields (Brown 1994). This isolation may have, in turn, allowed preventable patient suffering caused by a fragmented view of the patient's health care network. However, for the future, integration with other health professions is seen as mandatory in order to successfully address the education and practical implementation of health behavior change in the dental practice.

This realization has been the stimulus for the collaborative efforts initiated to write this book. Each of the co-authors has integrated the health behavior change principles in his or her clinical research agenda, patient care plans, or dental and dental hygiene curricula. The six subsequent chapters are uniquely aligned as a course to inspire and facilitate integration of health behavior change counselling in the dental practice.

Following this introduction, chapter 2 reveals "The Challenge of Behavior Change" and highlights the complexity of behavior change counselling in a clinical setting. Within chapter 3, "Communication and Health Behavior Change Counselling," the importance of establishing a good rapport is introduced together with the styles and key skills for effective communication. Subsequently, chapter 4 focuses on "Motivational Interviewing (MI) and Its Basic Tools" for use to engage the patient in discussion about behavior change. In chapter 5, "Brief Interventions in Promoting Health Behavior Change," several approaches on how to engage the patient in a short amount of time are introduced. In order to demonstrate the "Implementation of Health Behavior Change Principles in Dental Practice," chapter 6 presents the translation of the theory into practice. It presents a case scenario adapted for the dental practice. Chapter 7, "Health Behavior Change Education," discusses the implementation of health behavior change counselling into the dental and dental hygiene curriculum.

The theoretical content presented in this book provides more than sufficient background for the implementation of health behavior change counselling into practice. The reader may prefer to follow each chapter in sequence or utilize the key points provided at the beginning of each chapter to locate specific information.

REFERENCES

Berg, J., L.S. Evangelista, et al. (2006). Compliance. In: I.M. Lubkin and P.D. Larsen, *Chronic Illness: Impact and Interventions*. Sudbury, MA: Jones and Bartlett, 221–252.

Brown, L.F. (1994). Research in dental health education and health promotion: A review of the literature. *Health Educ Q* 21(1):83–102.

Chin, P.A. (2006). Change agent. In: I.M. Lubkin and P.D. Larsen, *Chronic Illness: Impact and Interventions*. Sudbury, MA: Jones and Bartlett, 323–350.

Gift, H.C., and B.A. White (1997). Health behavior research and oral health. In: D.S. Gochman, *Handbook of Health Behavior Research, IV: Relevance for Professionals and Issues for the Future*. New York: Plenum Press, 121–142.

Gochman, D.S. (1997). Relevance of health behavior research. *Handbook of Health Behavior Research, IV: Relevance for Professionals and Issues for the Future*. New York: Plenum Press, 377–393.

Larsen, P.D., P.R. Lewis, et al. (2006). Illness behavior and roles. In: I.M. Lubkin and P.D. Larsen, *Chronic Illness: Impact and Interventions*. Sudbury, MA: Jones and Bartlett, 23–44.

Rankin, S.H., K.D. Stallings, et al. (2005). Staff development in patient education. *Patient Education in Health and Illness*. Philadelphia: Lippincott Williams & Wilkins, 100–131.

Redman, B.K. (2007). The practice of patient education: Overview, motivation and learning. *The Practice of Patient Education: A Case Study Approach*. St. Louis: Mosby, 1–25.

World Health Organization (WHO). (2003). *Adherence to Long-Term Therapies: Evidence for Action*. Geneva, Switzerland: World Health Organization.

CHAPTER 2

THE CHALLENGE OF BEHAVIOR CHANGE

Nina Gobat, Vanessa Bogle, and Claire Lane

Key Points of This Chapter

- Behavior change is complex and can seem like a struggle for both the patient and the clinician.
- Patient behavior change happens outside the treatment room within the context of your patients' lives.
- There are ways of approaching the challenge of health behavior change that make it less stressful for the clinician and with a greater potential for effecting results in a brief period of time.
- There are limits to what you can achieve with advice alone: research suggests that the conversational environment in which the advice is given makes a significant difference to how that advice is received.
- Ambivalence—or "feeling two ways about something"—is a normal part of the change process.
- How you communicate with your patient makes all the difference: evidence has shown that the expression of empathy is perhaps the most important factor in facilitating patient behavior change.
- It will be the patient's task to say how and why he or she should or might change. The clinician's role is to elicit these arguments for change from the patient.
- For patients facing the need for a number of changes to be made, involving them in the process of decision making at the beginning is important. The use of a specific skill, agenda setting, and agreeing on priorities can facilitate this process.
- There are many different models and theories of behavior change that can help guide ways of thinking about practice.

INTRODUCTION

Behavior change requires effort. It involves consciously making different choices or adopting new habits and lifestyle patterns and is seldom comfortable, easy, or convenient. Consider the case of Mrs. K, a 38-year-old mother of three children. She comes home from a recent appointment with her dentist with a firm resolve to follow the self-care advice given. As the weeks pass, however, she loses momentum and one evening while halfheartedly flossing her teeth, she notices her gums bleeding more than usual. She feels guilty about this and so considers cancelling her upcoming dental hygiene appointment, not wanting to explain the increase in the bleeding of her gums to her hygienist.

We may agree that the worst step Mrs. K can take at this stage is to cancel her dental hygiene appointment. A basic understanding of the progression of gum disease would indicate that doing so is counterproductive. So, what happened to Mrs. K that she was considering taking a step like this? And further, how can dental clinicians encourage patients to make better decisions in support of the oral care they need?

Questions about how and why people act in certain ways in relation to their health have absorbed clinicians and behavioral scientists alike across many disciplines for years. Within the study of health behavior, many theories have been proposed and numerous studies conducted in an attempt to develop and evaluate effective interventions promoting behavior change. Theories vary in their philosophy of which factors determine behavior change. Some place greater emphasis on individual factors such as cognitions or emotions, while others include environmental factors such as socio-economic status or the influence of the family. However, the evidence to date suggests that behavior change is a challenging task and no single approach guarantees success.

In this chapter, we will focus on the challenge of addressing behavior change with patients at an individual level. First we will highlight some key concepts related to behavior change illustrated from both the patient's and the clinician's perspectives. We will then provide an overview of popular theories and models as ways of understanding behavior change.

BEHAVIOR CHANGE: SOME KEY CONCEPTS

This is a book for clinicians. The challenge of behavior change we will focus on lies within the oral health care environment. Clinicians say things like, "I repeat the same information every time I see this patient, what part of it doesn't he understand?" Patients say things like, "I've smoked for 25 years and now even my dentist is telling me to quit. Give me a break!" And the struggle continues.

So what is it about behavior change that gives rise to these challenges? One way to approach this question would be to have a look at the process of change itself and identify some key concepts. The following case example is an illustration of one man's struggles to improve his health. The story may have obvious parallels with patients you see in your practice. We will use this example to highlight some key concepts in working with behavior change in the clinic.

> Behavior change is complex and can seem like a struggle for both the patient and the clinician.

The patient's perspective

Consider a 65-year-old man receiving treatment for periodontal disease. This man is mostly compliant with his oral hygiene routine and attends his appointments regularly. However, despite repeated information and advice given to him by his dental clinician and others, he continues to smoke forty cigarettes a day. He is also slightly overweight and, on assessment, admitted he had a high sugar diet with little intention of changing this.

Several years into treatment the man returns for an appointment having lost a significant amount of weight. His dental clinician notes an improvement in his disease progression and asks the man what has changed. She learns that the man had started walking daily with his wife, who had recently retired. Encouraged by the success of losing some weight, he had made some small changes to his diet and had been steadily cutting down the amount he was smoking.

Clearly, stopping smoking and making some dietary changes significantly improved this man's general health as well as his periodontal condition. Of course the dental practitioner knew this and had been wanting him to make these changes for some time. However, this patient's perspective tells a different story. The man knew the benefits of quitting smoking but, despite efforts made in the past, he had not managed to succeed and had lost the confidence that this was something he was able to do. He would then try changing his diet. Results here were familiar too. He would start with the best intentions and then old habits would creep back in. Although he knew these changes would make a difference to his periodontal disease, he focused his efforts on his oral hygiene routine and attending visits and felt he was doing all he could to manage his oral health. His decision to start walking had very little to do with improving his oral health and more to do with joining his wife for walks, then feeling motivated by the effects of this activity. The man was encouraged by his dental clinician's response to these changes and this strengthened his resolve to maintain the changes further.

What does this simple story illustrate about behavior change?

Change can happen naturally in everyday life

It is now generally accepted that in many different contexts, positive change occurs relatively frequently without more formal intervention. One way of understanding behavior change interventions, therefore, is to see them as ways of facilitating this naturally occurring process (Miller and Rollnick 2002). Reflecting on this patient's story, we see that this man made changes at a time that made sense to him and in a way that made the effort seem worthwhile. A simple conclusion is this: that all patients have the potential to make changes despite the struggles that so frequently characterize this task. Reminding yourself of this potential can encourage you to approach the challenge of behavior change with optimism and curiosity, thereby creating a conversational environment more conducive to talk about change.

Intrinsic motivation affects patient behavior

There is a difference between motivation that arises from an internal source (intrinsic motivation) versus that which is prompted from an external source (extrinsic motivation). Take a moment to think about your own experience of change. There is a difference between your doing something because you decide it is a good idea and your doing something to receive a reward or to avoid punishment.

Intrinsic motivation is related to individual experiences of confidence, vitality, and self-esteem, and these factors are unique to each individual (Deci and Ryan 1985). Gaining an understanding of what these factors might be for your patient contributes to knowing how best to tap in to his or her positive potential for change.

Let us return to the story of the patient described above to illustrate this. The man in the example developed an inner sense of satisfaction and

THE CHALLENGE OF BEHAVIOR CHANGE

well-being not only due to the health improvements he was noticing but also as a result of the quality time he was spending with his wife. These internal factors reflect the man's intrinsic motivation to sustain the positive changes he had made and even begin to provoke some small changes in other areas of his life.

People change when they are ready

What happened to inspire the man in the case study to cut down on his smoking and change his diet? One way of answering this question would be to say that he simply reached a point when he was ready to make some changes. This concept of readiness was introduced with the Stages of Change model (Prochaska and DiClemente 1983) and plays a central role in helping us understand how it is that some patients seem "more motivated" to make changes than others. Motivation is a dynamic concept. At any one moment in time, patients may be at varying points of readiness to change a particular behavior. Additionally, they will be at different points of readiness for different behaviors. From the case study above, we can see that the man first made changes to his oral hygiene routine, then to his physical activity levels, to his diet, and, finally, to his tobacco use. From a "readiness" perspective, it seems clear that the man was "more ready" to comply with his oral health routine than with smoking cessation advice. Attempts by the clinician to influence his smoking behavior may therefore have been unsuccessful. And this would not have been because the man is generally "difficult" or "unmotivated."

Ambivalence is part of the process

Perhaps one of the greater limitations of behavior change theories proposed thus far is an over-reliance on logic or linear processes when approaching the change process (Ryan and Deci 2000). Behavior change appears, by nature, to be irrational. Attempts in this area are typically characterized by periods of success and then reverting back to familiar habits. Rather than being pathological in any way, this kind of process is both familiar and to be expected. Moreover, it can be captured succinctly with the concept of ambivalence.

Ambivalence is an internal process where a person feels two ways about doing something. Most people will experience a certain amount of ambivalence throughout the process of change (Rollnick et al. 2007; Ryan and

Deci 2000). The man in this case study clearly knew the reported health benefits of stopping smoking. His inability to quit smoking was not linked to a lack of information but rather to an internal "tug of war" where one part of him felt it important to do something about his smoking, that is, his early attempts to quit, but another part of him felt the task was too difficult. In addition to this, the man may have experienced some benefits to smoking. He may, for example, have felt that cigarettes helped him relax. No matter how illogical this may seem from the outside, when it comes to behavior, it is the patient's perception that counts toward what choices he or she will make.

Change happens in the context of our patients' lives

> Patient behavior change happens outside the treatment room within the context of our patients' lives.

This story illustrates a final key point: that patient behavior change happens outside the treatment room within the context of our patients' lives. Clinicians who take time to engage with their patients, listening closely to understand their life context, are certainly more likely to influence some of the decisions and choices their patients may make when leaving the consulting room.

The clinician's perspective

> There are ways of approaching the challenge of health behavior change that make it less stressful for the clinician and with a greater potential for effecting results in a brief period of time.

The clinician working with the man described above may tell a very different story. Every time they met the clinician would raise the subject of the patient's tobacco use, giving him information leaflets and a helpline number to help him with the recommendations provided. The man would sit and listen to the advice and take the leaflet home with him, but he seemed reluctant to talk about his tobacco use in any detail. At times he seemed irritable and sullen whenever the topic was brought up again. The clinician felt frustrated by this, as it was clear the man was making good attempts with his oral hygiene routine. It seemed impossible to understand why he couldn't grasp the improvements he could make by simply cutting down his tobacco consumption. The clinician would also give the man some information regarding diet but felt tobacco cessation was the greater priority.

This type of experience is fairly common in routine clinical practice. As a dental clinician, in any consultation, you may have as little as 5 or 10 minutes to speak with your patient about changes they could be making to improve their oral health. The frustrations expressed by the clinician working with this man are therefore understandable. However, there are ways of approaching this challenge that make it less stressful for the clinician and with a greater potential for effecting results in a brief period of time. The challenge remains to use the time available to maximum effect and to make the "window of opportunity" you have available count (see chapter 5).

Limitations of giving advice

A familiar approach in addressing oral health–related behavior change has been to give advice or to try to persuade patients toward a particular course of action. However, the limitation of this approach becomes clear when considering the psychological theory of reactance (Brehm 1966; Brehm and Brehm 1981). When someone feels pressured to accept a certain view or attitude, his or her immediate emotional reaction is to argue for the opposite. This reaction occurs when individuals perceive a freedom, or choice, is to be taken from them. As a result, trying to persuade a person to adopt a particular course of action frequently elicits the exact opposite result to the one you are trying to achieve.

> There are limits to what you can achieve with advice alone: research suggests that the conversational environment in which the advice is given makes a significant difference to how that advice is received.

This goes some way to explain why it is that traditional educational interventions have not proved effective in promoting patient behavior change (Renz et al. 2007). This is not to say that clinicians should not give advice or information to patients. However, research suggests that the conversational environment in which the advice is given makes a significant difference to how that advice is received (Salter et al. 2007). This finding complements research by Najavits and co-workers that emphasizes interpersonal interaction as the single most important factor in influencing motivation and behavior change (Najavits et al. 2000).

Another way of saying this is that it is the way in which we communicate with our patients that affects behavior change outcomes (Rollnick et al. 2007).

The role of ambivalence

Ambivalence—or "feeling two ways about something"—is a normal part of the change process.

A common assumption when working with motivation and behavior change is that this is a static or absolute concept. However, as discussed above, patients are seldom 100% certain about making a change or following recommended advice, even if this is clearly in the interest of improving their health. How might this appear to the clinician?

Take, for example, a patient who says:

> "I really want to floss properly in the evening but it seems to take too long."

If you recognize this as a statement of ambivalence you are likely to respond in a very different way than if you felt your patient was trying to explain why he or she doesn't floss. Likewise in the example given at the start of this section, the man may have tried to explain his struggle with stopping smoking to the clinician, only to be met with more information that he already knew. This would only have strengthened the patient's frustration, as well as the frustration of the clinician.

Changing behavior may be a struggle. However, clinicians who are skilled enough to help patients understand this struggle are clearly better equipped to help them resolve it. Recognizing ambivalence allows the clinician to respond to it in a more helpful way (Rollnick et al. 2007).

For example, compare the following two dialogues:

> Patient: "Every time I come here you give me these leaflets. I know I should stop smoking but I've done it for years and it's just not that easy." (Patient is expressing ambivalence)
> Clinician: "All the information you need to help you is on the leaflets I've given you. I'd suggest you give it a try." (Clinician responds giving advice and more information)

Now, compare with this dialogue below in which the clinician acknowledges ambivalence about behavior change:

Patient: "Every time I come here you give me these leaflets. I know I should stop smoking but I've done it for years and it's just not that easy." (Patient is expressing ambivalence)

Clinician: "You're ambivalent about this. Quitting smoking is harder than it seems. On the other hand you know the harm smoking causes to your health and you'd like to do something about it." (Clinician provides statement reflecting the patient's ambivalence)

In this second example, the clinician demonstrates an understanding of the patient's challenge and offers him a new way of seeing it himself. The patient is now more likely to respond non-defensively. Recognizing ambivalence as a normal part of the change process allows the clinician to create a conversational environment in which behavior change can be discussed constructively.

Interpersonal skills—a key clinical tool

In a busy clinical practice in which clinicians are faced with competing priorities and demands, it is not surprising that frustration is expressed toward patients who seem unwilling to make the necessary changes to support their treatment. However, we know that the attitude a clinician has toward a patient influences behavioral outcomes (Miller and Rollnick 2002; Rogers 1951; Rollnick et al. 2007). Behavior change is a subtle and confounding process. It is essential that the patient feels heard and understood. Empathy is a key skill in being able to communicate this to patients. Change takes conscious effort and is a process characterized by periods of successes and periods of relapse (DiClemente 2003). Empathy is a skill that enables clinicians to accurately reflect back to patients both the content and emotions underlying what they have said. It plays a key role in enabling clinicians to swiftly and effectively communicate their understanding of this process, thereby influencing behavioral outcomes.

How you communicate with your patient makes all the difference: evidence has shown that the expression of empathy is perhaps the most important factor in facilitating patient behavior change.

One review has shown that the use of interpersonal skills such as expression of empathy is perhaps the most important factor in facilitating patient behavior change (Najavits et al. 2000). It is the clinician's "way of being" with patients that has a significant influence on how motivated they are to change. In addition, as patients are all different, clinicians need to be flexible in the way that they consult with patients to increase their motivation. This concept of flexible communication styles in practice, rather than a fixed way of consulting, is something that has been advocated by Rollnick and co-workers (Rollnick et al. 2007). By matching their consulting style to the behavioral style of the patient, clinicians can select the "way of being" most appropriate to facilitate change for that patient.

Limitations of a "fix it" approach

A common approach for the clinician to address the challenge of behavior change is to assume that patients are somehow lacking in something. If they had enough knowledge, insight, skills, or concern about their disease, then they would make a change (Morrison and Bennett 2005). This way of thinking leads clinicians to logically assume that if they were just to give patients the knowledge they seem to lack, then patients would change. So clinicians respond by giving patients information and advice or repeatedly teaching them the skills needed to be adherent, sometimes with an increasing sense of urgency. However, unlike a restorative dental procedure such as filling a cavity, behavior change interventions do not necessarily work with the same laws of cause and effect. In addition, behavior does not occur in an isolated manner divorced from the everyday demands and expectations of an individual's life. Instead, it calls for a different way of approaching the challenge and another, sometimes opposite way of thinking about it.

> It will be the patient's task to say how and why he or she should or might change. The clinician's role is to elicit these arguments for change from the patient.

The logic behind many of the approaches in this book is that there is another way of looking at this; it is the patient's task to say how and why they should or might change. The clinician's role is to elicit these arguments for change from the patient. Terry Pratchett, a British author, humorously describes this with a touch of irony in the following quote: "After all, when you seek advice from someone it's certainly not because you want them to give it. You just want them to be there while you talk to yourself" (Pratchett 1997). This is also the premise of Self-Perception Theory (Bem 1967), which holds that it is the individual's perception of his or her difficulties that has the most powerful effect in persuading one to change. Another way of saying this is, "As I hear myself speak, I learn what I believe and it is persuasive to me because I said it."

Agreeing on priorities

Finally, as illustrated in the case study earlier, you may be working with a patient for whom there are a number of potential behavior change areas, with competing priorities. The man in this example was faced with making a number of changes: (1) complying with his oral hygiene routine, (2) changing his smoking, and (3) changing his diet. The clinician working with him may have felt that smoking cessation was the priority area to work on. However, adopting the patient's point of view, he identified a different place to start. Involving patients in the process of decision making at the beginning is important. The use of a specific skill, agenda setting, can facilitate this process (Rollnick et al. 2007). You can find out more about agenda setting in chapter 3.

> For patients facing the need for a number of changes to be made, involving them in the process of decision making at the beginning is important. The use of a specific skill, agenda setting, and agreeing on priorities can facilitate this process.

UNDERSTANDING HEALTH BEHAVIOR CHANGE

Numerous approaches to explaining behavior change have been proposed in an attempt to provide a framework upon which health behavior change interventions can be based (Deci and Ryan 1985). We will now move on to provide an overview of some popular models and theories of behavior change, some of which provide the foundation to more practical approaches described in detail throughout this book (see chapters 4 and 5).

> There are many different models and theories of behavior change that can help guide ways of thinking about practice.

Social cognitive theory and self-efficacy theory

Social Cognitive Theory is associated with the work of Albert Bandura. Bandura's early work was strongly influenced by theories of social learning and imitation described in 1941 by Miller and Dollard (Miller and Dollard 1941). However, by the late 1970s, Bandura identified a key missing element: self-efficacy (Bandura 1997). Self-efficacy beliefs reflect an internal awareness that one is able to perform a specific task. Without an internal belief that one is able to make a change, change is unlikely to happen. In this way, Bandura proposed a view of human behavior in which the beliefs that people have about themselves are central to the choices they make in shaping their lives.

A brief diversion to the world of clinical practice illustrates how this understanding can influence clinicians. Consider if patients tell you:

> "I just can't floss the way you want me to."

They may be expressing low self-efficacy in their ability to floss. Having confidence in one's ability to do something is more than having the skills to be able to do it. It is also about an internal belief that one is able to make a change and integrate this change into everyday habits and routines with ease. Recognizing this statement as one indicating low self-efficacy would enable the clinician to respond in a way that might in fact increase confidence, therefore leading to an effective outcome (Rollnick et al. 2007). Chapter 4 explores this in more detail when discussing self-efficacy in the context of Motivational Interviewing (Miller and Rollnick 2002), and chapter 6 offers practical examples of how this appears in the clinical arena.

Bandura's Social Cognitive Theory embraced the concept of self-efficacy and considered the role of the environment in shaping human behavior (Bandura 1997). This theory suggests that environmental factors such as socio-economic status and familial structure are significant in the way they impact self-efficacy beliefs and aspirations. With this view, an individual is both a product of the environment and active in influencing the environment through the choices he or she makes. Bandura's work had a profound influence on psychological thinking and on subsequent theories of behavior change.

The health belief model

The health belief model (Figure 2.1) attempts to explain and predict health behaviors by focusing on the attitude and beliefs of individuals (Becker and Maiman 1975). The model hypotheses that an individual's decision to change behavior is determined primarily by two elements: one's perception of a threat to personal health, and one's perception of the efficacy of treatment proposed to reduce the threat. An individual's perception of a threat is determined by two underlying beliefs, namely the perceived susceptibility of the disease and the perceived severity or seriousness of the disease. The perceived efficacy of

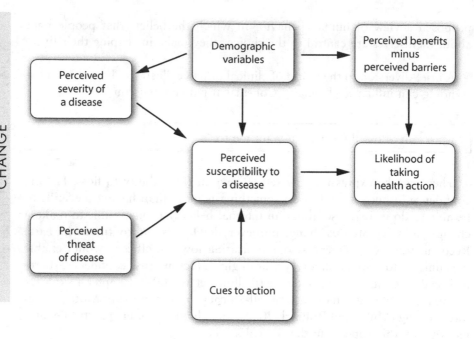

Figure 2.1. The health belief model (Becker and Maiman 1975).

treatment is dependant on the individual's assessment of the benefits and barriers to performing the suggested behavior. Further dimensions were added to later versions of the model, namely health motivation (motivation to be concerned about health matters), perceived efficacy (the belief in one's ability to successfully enact a desired behavior to produce desired outcomes), and cues to action (events that motivate people to take action). Other variables including demographics (gender) and psychological characteristics (personality and peer group pressure) were also included.

The health belief model highlights the importance of the individual's subjective reality. For example, if a patient believes that flossing is not an essential part of good oral hygiene and doesn't see this as threatening his or her health in any way, he or she is unlikely to see a need for changing an oral hygiene routine. In the context of this model, information and advice is therefore only helpful if it is meaningful to an individual and is assimilated into his or her belief and value system.

The health belief model has been used to guide research, and support for the theory has been demonstrated. However, its relevance within oral health–related contexts has been debated in the literature. For example, Weisenberg and co-workers conducted a school-based, preventive dentistry study with 11- to 14-year-olds using the health belief model to predict and understand their long-term oral health behavior (Weisenberg et al. 1980). The authors concluded that changing health beliefs of children to achieve acceptance of preventive health procedures such as fluoride treatments is difficult and often unrelated to behavior. In addition, they found an inverse relationship between health beliefs and behavior through consistently finding that lower beliefs of susceptibility led to greater program acceptance than higher beliefs of susceptibility.

Theory of planned behavior

Social psychologists Fishbein and Ajzen developed the theory of reasoned action, a theory linking a person's attitude with his or her behavior. This theory was later expanded and developed into the theory of planned behavior (Ajzen 1985) by adding a further construct to the earlier model to enhance its ability to predict more complex non-volitional behaviors. This third dimension, perceived behavioral control, is similar to Bandura's concept of self-efficacy. It considers the importance of perceptions of control over performance of the behavior as a further predictor of behavior.

The theory of planned behavior (Figure 2.2) proposes that the best predictor of behavior is an individual's intention (the construct representing motivation) to perform the behavior. The three components influencing intention are

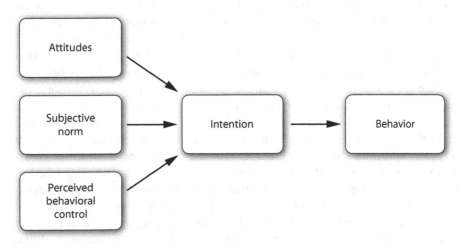

Figure 2.2. Theory of planned behavior (Ajzen 1985).

1. attitudes toward the behavior: an individual's positive/negative evaluation of performing the behavior;

2. subjective norms associated with the behavior: an individual's perception of the social pressures exerted on him or her to perform or not perform the behavior; and

3. perceived behavioral control: the degree to which the individual perceives the behavior to be under his or her control. This component is said to reflect external factors (e.g., social support and time) and internal factors (e.g., skill, self-efficacy). It is suggested that it can also directly influence behavior when the behavior is not under the complete control of the individual.

The efficacy of the theory of planned behavior in explaining intention and behavior has been widely examined to predict a range of health behaviors (Conner and Sparkes 1996). The findings generally support this theory in its ability to predict intention. However, evidence suggests it is less effective in predicting actual behavior change and is, therefore, limited in enabling clinicians to effectively influence behavior change outcomes with patients.

The transtheoretical model of behavior change

The transtheoretical model (TTM) emerged as an attempt to integrate approaches in addiction treatment (DiClemente 2003). Early research on TTM consisted of naturalistic studies of people's attempts to stop smoking. As the research broadened, the model developed to capture the nature of the process of change across a number of dimensions. The TTM proposes that individuals pass through five main stages when attempting to change behavior (Figure 2.3). The process is dynamic and individuals may cycle through the stages several times in their efforts to change, or they may remain at a stage for some time without movement. Each of the stages is defined by specific tasks that individuals need to complete in order to move through to the next stage. In addition, the model incorporates a set of ten processes that create and sustain movement through the stages. These processes are described in two categories: cognitive or experiential (e.g., commitment to act or believing in the ability to do so) and behavioral (e.g., being open and trusting to someone about \problems). The model also describes signposts or markers of change. Finally, it considers the context of change (DiClemente 2003; Prochaska and DiClemente 1983, 1989). The TTM explains the process of

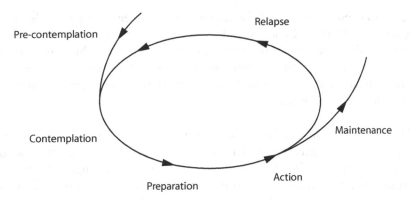

Figure 2.3. The transtheoretical model of behavior change (TTM; Prochaska and DiClemente 1983).

change through observation of the interaction between these four dimensions (i.e., stages, processes, markers, and contexts of change). Interventions to facilitate movement through the stage cycle have been proposed through matching the intervention to the particular stage an individual is in.

The first of the five stages described is that of pre-contemplation. Persons in this stage do not consider their behavior—such as smoking or non-compliance with oral hygiene routines—to be affecting their health negatively in any way. They do not see any reason why they should consider changing their behavior despite any objective evidence that may be shown to contradict this. Stage two is the stage of contemplation, in which patients have become aware that a problem exists and begin to contemplate change. They typically vacillate between change and no change, both in their thinking and what they actually do. As part of this process, they may weigh up the pros and cons of change. Once patients begin to get ready for change, they move into stage three, the stage of preparation. Patients in this stage have the clear intention to change their behavior and begin to make small changes in this direction. Smokers in this phase might, for example, cut back on smoking or not buy a carton of cigarettes but rather one pack at a time. These patients may not have integrated the change of behavior fully into their lives but are beginning to take some steps toward doing so. Prochaska and co-workers refer to this stage as the phase of decision making (Prochaska et al. 1992). Patients are understood to have made a decision to change and are beginning to formulate ways of following this through. Stage four is the stage of action, in which patients are actively engaged in the changed behavior. They might have stopped smoking, be flossing regularly, or begun drinking sugar-free drinks. Permanent behavior change takes some time to integrate, however, and is

THE CHALLENGE OF BEHAVIOR CHANGE

unlikely to occur right away. The action phase is often a time of high motivation where patients feel encouraged by their success. However, this is also a time when they are vulnerable to relapse back into old habits and patterns. With sustained efforts and support, patients move into the final stage, maintenance, during which the new behavior is more fully integrated into their lifestyle habits and routines.

The TTM has come under criticism in recent years, with particular regard to rejecting the stage-based model on conceptual grounds. Critics argue that the model oversimplifies the complexities of behavior change into artificial, discrete categories based on arbitrary cut-off points (Davidson 1992, 1998). West elaborated on some of the flaws of the TTM and argued strongly for it to be discarded on the grounds that it has impeded the advancement of health promotion (West 2005). Davidson's critique of the TTM also pointed out numerous problems with the model but concluded that despite these, the model continued to have heuristic and practical utility, in the addictions field at least (Davidson 1998).

Self-determination theory

Self-determination theory developed out of studies into the results of environmental effects on intrinsic motivation (Markland et al. 2005). Motivation is fundamental to all human behavior and central to self-regulation. It can be defined as a force that directs and energizes behavior and encompasses personality factors, social variables, and cognitions. Understanding motivation is of paramount importance to clinicians involved in helping their clients to act (Ryan and Deci 2000). The results of meta-analyses suggest that individuals are motivated by situations where some choice, control, and self-determination exists, and they prefer not to be controlled and pressured (Koestner et al. 2002). However, the presence of motivation may be insufficient on its own to ensure behavioral change.

Self-determination theory is a general theory of human motivation and personality that explains differences in motivation. It is made up of four mini-theories, each of which has been developed to explain a set of motivationally based phenomena. The theory is concerned with conditions that elicit and sustain intrinsic motivation. It proposes that individuals (regardless of gender, group, or culture) have an innate psychological need to act in autonomous, self-determined ways and to engage in tasks that are intrinsically meaningful, as opposed to those that are mandated by internal or external forces. Deci and Ryan examined factors related to intrinsically motivated behavior and identified three key innate psychological needs essential for health and well-being (Deci and Ryan 1985).

1. Competence: Perceived competence in the ability to enact the necessary behavior to yield the desired outcomes.

2. Autonomy: Related to self-determination and refers to feelings of perceived behavioral control and to feelings that one is voluntarily engaging in the behavior, regardless of whether the behavior is dependent on others or not.

3. Relatedness: Strive for positive interactions with other people. Considered the most fundamental psychological need; developmental studies have found that relatedness is essential for growth of autonomy functioning.

However, if social factors do not allow for the satisfaction of these three needs, the model suggests that this will result in diminished motivation, impaired psychological development, alienation, and possibly poor performance (Deci and Ryan 1991).

One example of a well-designed study of self-determination theory applied to dental practice is that by Münster Halvari and Halvari (Münster Halvari and Halvari 2006). These authors developed an intervention and tested it by randomly allocating eighty-six participants to either receive the intervention or to receive "standard dental care" (as a control group). Self-determination theory was translated into practice through particular strategic steps. In delivering the intervention, clinicians began by asking the patients about what they perceived their dental problem to be. They then listened and acknowledged the patient's feelings before providing highly personalized information and presenting a range of different treatment options, emphasizing the patient's right to choose to adopt these treatments or not. When demonstrating brushing and flossing, the clinician allowed the patient to practice the behaviors and reinforced the patient's ability to conduct these practices well. However, clinicians did not put the patient under pressure to conform to these practices, leaving the choice about whether to continue up to the patient.

Patients who received this intervention demonstrated a greater sense of perceived competence and self-motivation than those who received standard care, as measured using validated instruments over the 7-month study period. Patients in the intervention group also showed a significantly greater decrease in plaque and gingivitis in comparison to those in the control group. In addition, they showed better dental self-care and more positive dental health attitudes in comparison to controls. The authors conclude that the use of an "autonomy-supportive approach" can positively influence patient self-determination and motivation.

Self-determination theory offers a theoretical framework for understanding the processes involved in motivating people to change. Parallels have been drawn in the understanding of human motivation between this theory and Motivational Interviewing, a scientific method of facilitating behavior change (Markland et al. 2005) described in chapter 4 of this book. It is suggested that self-determination theory could be seen to provide a theoretical framework in attempting to understand the efficacy of Motivational Interviewing. However, it is worth bearing in mind that many have questioned the cross-cultural validity of this model, particularly its emphasis on autonomy. This is because not all cultures have an emphasis on the self as an individual.

SUMMARY

Human behavior is complex and confounding. Understanding the best way to influence it presents a challenge to clinicians working in oral health–related contexts. From a review of the theoretical foundations of behavior and behavior change, it is evident that there is no single way to address this challenge. However, there are some clear and practical guidelines for clinicians introduced in this chapter and expanded upon throughout this book. Encouraging patients to speak about solutions they identify themselves and placing them in the role of an active decision maker, free of coercion, may be important. Helping patients feel confident about making changes may also play a useful role. Taking time to establish a good relationship with patients and switching consulting style in line with the patient's needs is perhaps the single most important thing that clinicians can do, on an individual level, to influence motivation. In short, this is about effective communication.

REFERENCES

Ajzen, I. (1985). From intentions to action: A theory of planned behavior. In: J. Kuhl and J. Beckman, *Action Control: From Cognitions to Behaviors*. New York: Springer, 11–39.

Bandura, A. (1997). *Self-Efficacy: The Exercise of Control*. New York: W.H. Freeman.

Becker, M.H., and L.A. Maiman. (1975). Sociobehavioral determinants of compliance with health and medical care recommendations. *Med Care* 13(1):10–24.

Bem, D.J. (1967). Self-perception: An alternative interpretation of cognitive dissonance phenomena. *Psychol Rev* 74(3):183–200.

Brehm, J.W. (1966). *A Theory of Psychological Reactance*. New York: Academic Press.

Brehm, S.S., and J.W. Brehm (eds.). (1981). *Psychological Reactance: A Theory of Freedom and Control*. New York: Academic Press.

Conner, M., and P. Sparkes. (1996). The theory of planned behaviour and health behaviours. In: M. Conner and P. Norman, *Predicting Health Behaviour*. Buckingham, UK: Open University Press, 121–162.

Davidson, R. (1992). Prochaska and DiClemente's model of change: A case study? *Br J Addict* 87:821–822.

Davidson, R. (1998) The transtheoretical model: a critical overview. In: *Treating Addictive Behaviors*, 2nd edn, Miller, W. and Heather, N. eds, pp. 25–38. Plenum Press, London.

Deci, E.L., and R.M. Ryan (eds.). (1985). *Intrinsic Motivation and Self Determination in Human Behaviour*. New York: Plenum Press.

Deci, E.L. and R.M. Ryan. (1991). A motivational approach to self: Integration in personality. In: *Perspectives on Motivation*, R. Dienstbier, p. 237–288. Lincoln, Neb.: University of Nebraska Press.

DiClemente, C.C. (ed.). (2003). *Addiction and Change: How Addictions Develop and Addicted People Recover*. New York: Guilford Press.

Koestner, R., N. Lekes, et al. (2002). Attaining personal goals: Self-concordance plus implementation intentions equals success. *J Personality Social Psychology* 83(1):231–244.

Markland, D., R.M. Ryan, et al. (2005). Motivational interviewing and self-determination theory. *J Social Clinical Psychology* 24(6):811–831.

Miller, N.E., and J. Dollard (eds.). (1941). *Social Learning and Imitation*. London: Oxford University Press.

Miller, W.R., and S. Rollnick (eds.). (2002). *Motivational Interviewing: Preparing People for Change*, 2nd ed. New York: Guilford Press.

Morrison, V., and P. Bennett (eds.). (2005). *An Introduction to Health Psychology*. Harlow, England: Prentice Hall.

Münster Halvari, A.E., and H. Halvari. (2006). Motivational predictors of change in oral health: An experimental test of self-determination theory. *Motivation and Emotion* 30(4):295–306.

Najavits, L.M., P. Crits-Christoph, et al. (2000). Clinicians' impact on the quality of substance use disorder treatment. *Subst Use Misuse* 35(12–14):2161–2190.

Pratchett, T. (1997). *Jingo*. London: Victor Gollancz.

Prochaska, J.O., and C.C. DiClemente. (1983). Stages and processes of self-change of smoking: Toward an integrative model of change. *J Consult Clin Psychol* 51(3):390–395.

Prochaska, J.O., and C.C. DiClemente. (1989). Toward a comprehensive, transtheoretical model of change. In: W.R. Miller and N. Heather, *Treating Addictive Behaviours: Processes of Change*. New York: Plenum Press.

Prochaska, J.O., C.C. DiClemente, et al. (1992). In search of how people change: Applications to addictive behaviors. *Am Psychol* 47(9):1102–1114.

Renz, A., M. Ide, et al. (2007). Psychological interventions to improve adherence to oral hygiene instructions in adults with periodontal diseases. *Cochrane Database Syst Rev* (2), CD005097.

Rogers, C. (ed.). (1951). *Client Centred Therapy, Its Current Practice, Implications and Theory.* Boston: Houghton Mifflin.

Rollnick, S., W.R. Miller, et al. (eds.). (2007). *Motivational Interviewing in Health Care.* New York: Guilford Press.

Ryan, R.M., and E.L. Deci. (2000). Self-determination theory and the facilitation of intrinsic motivation, social development, and well-being. *Am Psychol* 55(1): 68–78.

Salter, C., R. Holland, et al. (2007). "I haven't even phoned my doctor yet." The advice giving role of the pharmacist during consultations for medication review with patients aged 80 or more: Qualitative discourse analysis. *Br Medical J* 334(7603):1101.

Weisenberg, M., S.S. Kegeles, et al. (1980). Children's health beliefs and acceptance of a dental preventive activity. *J Health Soc Behav* 21(1):59–74.

West, R. (2005). Time for a change: Putting the transtheoretical (Stages of Change) model to rest. *Addiction* 100(8):1036–1039.

THE CHALLENGE OF BEHAVIOR CHANGE

CHAPTER 3

COMMUNICATION AND HEALTH BEHAVIOR CHANGE COUNSELLING

Claire Lane

Key Points of This Chapter

- If the clinician is able to create an environment of understanding and respect for the patient's autonomy, the patient may feel more comfortable in discussing health behavior change. Good, skillful communication is the key to creating this kind of environment.
- Selecting the right style of communication for a given consultation is often the key to creating and maintaining a good rapport. Clinicians might communicate with their patients in daily practice, using either a directing, guiding, or following style.
- Four main communication skills can be used to implement a guiding style of communication with patients. These are summarized by the acronym OARS, which stands for "open questions," "affirmations," "reflective listening," and "summarizing."
- Open questions encourage patients to explore how they feel about a particular behavior and to describe how the behavior fits into their life. They help the clinician to gain a deeper understanding of a patient's views on change.
- Affirmations that demonstrate appreciation for the patient's efforts can be useful in helping the patient believe that he or she has the ability to change.
- Reflective listening enables the listener to check what he or she has understood from what the speaker has said. Moreover, it enables the speaker to feel understood.
- Before moving on in the dental visit it is important to summarize and demonstrate to the patient that the clinician has listened, understood, and taken on board what the patient has said.

INTRODUCTION

As was highlighted in chapter 2, the task of changing behavior is often complex and varies between individuals. Thus, the challenges raised concerning health behavior change affect both patients as well as clinicians.

There is often an assumption in clinical practice that if patients are not doing what is "good for them," then they must be lacking in knowledge. Although information and advice does have a place within many behavior change consultations, it is often patients' inner feelings about what change might mean for them that create perceived barriers to change, rather than a lack of information alone (Department of Health 2004). This signals a phenomenon known as *ambivalence*—having mixed feelings about change, and in turn feeling unsure or indecisive. Many people can think of a time in their lives when they have struggled to make a decision—where they have felt a sense of inner conflict about which course of action is the best choice, or a sense of hopelessness when neither path seems better than the other.

Many clinicians consult with ambivalent patients on a daily basis. It is often obvious that certain behaviors are damaging patients' oral health. Perhaps it is smoking or their diet that is causing most of the problems. Perhaps the patients are not following the oral hygiene regimen that has been recommended. Despite the number of times you have told them what they need to do, they never seem to do it. This may lead to the clinician feeling a number of different emotions—ranging from worry and concern, through to frustration and helplessness.

The main question we are left with then is how can the dental clinician address the complex task of health behavior change in a way that engages the patient to think about the issue, without triggering tension and resistance during the dental visit?

Traditionally, patients are passive recipients of information regarding how and why they should change their behavior. Individuals often feel more reluctant to think about change if they perceive their freedom is being compromised (Brehm 1966). So perhaps if the clinician is able to create an environment of understanding and respect for the patient's autonomy, a patient may feel more comfortable in discussing health behavior change.

COMMUNICATION AND HEALTH
BEHAVIOR CHANGE COUNSELLING

Good, skillful communication is the key to creating this kind of environment. Communication is a process by which we allocate and convey meanings in an attempt to create shared understanding with others. To that end, the choice of language, tone of voice, non-verbal cues, and gestures we use are important in ensuring the right message is conveyed. As highlighted in chapter 2, the way in which the patient is spoken to can make the difference between feeling that the clinician is helping him or her to change or feeling that he or she is being pushed into something the patient is not happy with. If the dental clinician can accurately select the most appropriate style of communication to employ in a given consultation, and utilize communication skills that make the patient feel respected and in control of any changes to be made, this will create a setting where a productive discussion about change can take place.

If the clinician is able to create an environment of understanding and respect for the patient's autonomy the patient may feel more comfortable in discussing health behavior change. Good, skillful communication is the key to creating this kind of environment.

THE RELATIONSHIP BETWEEN THE CLINICIAN AND THE PATIENT

The first initial step in any consultation about health behavior change should be to create a good "rapport" or "constructive relationship" with the patient. A good rapport will encourage the patient to be open and honest in the consultation. In contrast, a bad rapport may result in the patient just telling you what he or she believes you want to hear. Rapport is important to consider, as previous research has shown that the quality of the relationship between the clinician and the patient correlates with patient behavior change outcomes (Najavits et al. 2000).

Take a few moments to think about a person in your life with whom you feel at ease to talk. What is it about him or her that makes you feel comfortable? What kinds of things does he or she do?

In addition to your own ideas, there are some suggestions below that you might find helpful to consider when thinking about how to create a good rapport with your own patients.

Smile and welcome patients into appointments:

- Do they feel comfortable coming into the surgery?

- Have you seen them before?

- Do you know their names?

Think about the non-verbals:

- Have you taken off your mask, so patients can see your face when you are talking to them?

- Are patients sitting up when you are speaking to them?

- Are you giving patients your attention when they are speaking?

Think about when you ask questions:

- Can patients respond to you?

- Are you assuming what patients' responses would be?

Take some time to listen to patients:

- Why have they come along to see you today?

- What do they understand about their oral health?

- How do they feel about treatment?

- How do they feel about things they need to do to maintain their oral health?

Make them feel comfortable enough to come back in the future:

- Do you tell patients you look forward to seeing them again?

- Do patients feel they will be "told off" if they do come back?

Good communication reflects a good clinician-patient relationship, and in turn creates a good relationship. Selecting the right style of communication for a given consultation is often the key to creating and maintaining a good rapport.

COMMUNICATION AND HEALTH
BEHAVIOR CHANGE COUNSELLING

STYLES OF COMMUNICATION

In our daily lives there are a number of different styles we use when communicating with others. Rollnick and colleagues describe a simple three-style model for understanding how health care clinicians might communicate with their patients in daily practice, using either a directing, guiding, or following style (Rollnick et al. 2007).

> Selecting the right style of communication for a given consultation is often the key to creating and maintaining a good rapport. Clinicians might communicate with their patients in daily practice, using either a directing, guiding, or following style.

Directing

A *directing* style involves the delivery of expert advice and help. This has traditionally been the dominant approach within health care settings. Directing is best employed where there is a good rapport between the clinician and the patient. The information should be well-timed, personally relevant, and delivered in such a way as to engage the patient.

Following

A *following* style utilizes listening skills and occurs in situations where sensitivity is required (such as when a patient is upset). The goal of a clinician using a following style is not to solve the patient's problem immediately but to provide support and encouragement (for example, when breaking bad news to a patient).

Guiding

The third, more complex style described by Rollnick and co-workers is *guiding* (Rollnick et al. 2007). In guiding, the clinician and patient work together to help the patient identify his or her own goals and how he or she might best achieve them. This style is most appropriate when talking to patients about making health behavior changes—especially with those who may be ambivalent about changing.

It is important to note, however, that skilled judgment is required by the clinician in order to select which style is most appropriate for each situation. Consider what the consequences of sticking with one style might be. Consider also what might happen if the wrong style is used with a particular patient. Skilled clinical communication is about being able to effectively identify which styles of communication are best suited to a given point during the dental visit and being able to switch flexibly between those styles during the interaction.

When it comes to behavior change issues, some patients may require "direction"—particularly those who have stated that they want further information or advice. Others may have more pressing concerns—for example, after receiving some bad news during an examination—and need to be "followed." However, those patients who appear to know what they need to do but have not managed to do it yet may be more receptive to a "guiding" style (Rollnick et al. 2007).

A helpful exercise to consider which style might be more appropriate (directing, guiding, or following) is provided via the examples below:

> "What can I do to stop needing a filling every time I come back here?" (Directing)

> "I'm really afraid that I'm going to lose my teeth." (Following)

> "I can see how flossing might help my gums, but I just find it so difficult to fit in." (Guiding)

> "It would be really helpful to know what kind of foods I should avoid." (Directing)

> "I know that smoking isn't good for me, but it's the only pleasure I have in life." (Guiding)

> "There's so much going on in my life and now I have to worry about my teeth too?" (Following)

COMMUNICATION AND HEALTH
BEHAVIOR CHANGE COUNSELLING

It is important to be sensitive to the patient's reaction to a particular style of communication. If the rapport between you and the patient seems to be breaking down (the patient seems uncomfortable, disengaged, confused, or maybe resistant), this should be a sign that a particular style does not appear to be working. This can serve as a signal to the clinician that one might need to switch and try another style to get the rapport back on track.

KEY SKILLS FOR COMMUNICATING ABOUT HEALTH BEHAVIOR CHANGE

There are four main communication skills that can be used to implement a guiding style of communication with patients. These are summarized by the acronym OARS, which stands for "open questions," "affirmations," "reflective listening," and "summarizing." These may be terms that you are familiar with. Alternatively, you may not have encountered them before.

To effectively use a guiding style, it is important to incorporate OARS skillfully when communicating with patients about health behavior change. Using these skills helps the patient to feel understood, supported, encouraged, and able to get his or her point across. This is useful for the clinician, who can effectively do less, yet understand more about the patient's motivations for change.

In chapter 6, you will learn more about how OARS can be further refined during Motivational Interviewing to draw out a patient's intrinsic motivation. For now, however, we shall concentrate on using OARS to maintain a good rapport, have a productive discussion about health behaviors with a patient, and understand the patient's perspective on change.

There are six broad questions that need to be considered in relation to communicating about health behavior change. These are addressed in turn in the sections below, and illustrations of individual OARS skills, commensurate with a guiding style, are provided.

> Four main communication skills can be used to implement a guiding style of communication with patients. These are summarized by the acronym OARS, which stands for "open questions," "affirmations," "reflective listening," and "summarizing."

Question 1: Is the patient happy to talk with you about behavior change?

There are a number of consequences associated with talking with a patient who is not ready to engage in a discussion about his or her health behavior. At best, patients may simply decide that they will ignore what they are told; at worst, they can be argumentative or resistant. Individuals may even be at different stages of readiness to change different aspects of one health behavior (Rollnick et al. 1999). They may have a pressing issue that is more important for them to talk about that is affecting their readiness to change. To this end, the dental clinician should always ask permission to discuss health behavior with a patient, rather than just telling the patient that there will be a discussion about his or her health behavior. This can be achieved through asking a simple question, such as:

> "How would you feel about having a quick chat about your smoking this afternoon?"

Within clinical consultations, it is often the case that there is more than one health behavior affecting the patient's oral health. Achieving small changes can make a patient feel more able and confident to make other changes (Bandura 1995). In these situations, it is important to start where the patient feels most comfortable and encourage him or her to suggest what area he or she would like to talk about, rather than simply selecting what the dental clinician feels is the most pressing issue. Again, this can be addressed through a question such as:

> "There are a number of different things we could talk about today. I'm just wondering if there is anything related to your oral health that you would like to talk about?"

Agenda setting chart

One clinical tool that can help with this task is an "agenda setting chart" (Rollnick et al. 1999), an example of which can be seen in Figure 3.1.

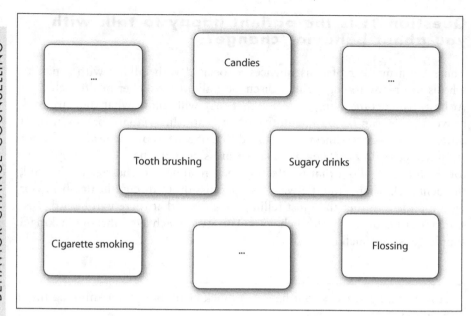

Figure 3.1. Agenda setting chart.

The agenda setting chart contains a number of shapes containing words for various issues in oral health and some blank shapes for other factors to be inserted by the patient. The patient then selects the issue that he or she would like to talk about first. The clinician should be prepared for the patient to raise issues that may not have been anticipated—for example, patients suffering with periodontitis may be more concerned about what the hereditary aspects of the condition might mean for their children, rather than their individual health, at that particular moment in time.

Deciding to talk about behavior change should ultimately be the patient's choice, to increase his or her feeling of personal freedom to make decisions, and in turn lower resistance (Brehm 1966). This can be achieved by

- inviting, not forcing, the patient to discuss behavior change,

- asking simple questions about the how the patient would feel to talk about behavior change, and

- if multiple issues need to be addressed, encouraging the patient to select the issue he or she feels most happy to talk about.

Question 2: How are you asking questions?

The amount of information collected and the degree of understanding achieved can be facilitated or inhibited by the kinds of questions that are asked. Therefore, it is important to consider whether the questions that are asked in the consultation are limiting the information available to you or encouraging the patient to provide the information required. It is here that the first of the OARS skills ("open questions") shall be discussed.

It is important at this point to distinguish the difference between a "closed question" and an "open question." Closed questions are those that encourage brief answers, whereas open questions encourage longer answers. For example, a closed question might be:

> "Do you floss every day?"

This limits the patient's response to "yes," "no," or "sometimes yes, sometimes no." Not only does this restrict the patient to a minimal response, it also means that the clinician has little insight as to why this may be the case. This makes it harder to discuss health behavior change in a way that is productive and helps the patient to consider change.

Open questions encourage the patient to explore how he or she feels about a particular behavior and describe how the behavior fits into his or her life. They help the clinician to gain a deeper understanding of the patient's views on change.

On the other hand, open questions allow for a more detailed response. For example, rather than asking:

> "Do you floss every day?"

an open question the clinician could ask is:

> "How do you feel about your flossing?"

When talking with a patient about behavior change, the clinician should use mainly open rather than closed questions. Looking at the example above, it is clear to see that asking:

> "How are you managing with your flossing?"

would provide the clinician with valuable information about the factors that affect how often the patient uses floss. Open questions encourage the patient to explore how he or she feels about a particular behavior and describe how the behavior fits into his or her life. They help the clinician to gain a deeper understanding of the patient's views on change. Closed questions only give limited information, which makes it harder for the clinician to deduce information that may be clinically relevant. This is not to say that closed questions should never be used. However, to build up an accurate picture of the issues affecting change, closed questions should be kept to a minimum to encourage this exploration.

In the following few examples, consider moving the closed questions into open questions:

"How many cigarettes do you smoke per day?"

"Do you drink a lot of fizzy soft drinks?"

"How long do you spend brushing your teeth?"

"Do you floss regularly?"

"Have you noticed that your gums are sore at all?"

Open questions are useful because they

- provide valuable clinical information that the clinician may not have anticipated,

- give the patient a chance to get his or her perspective across, enhancing the rapport within the consultation,

- provide an insight into the factors affecting change,

- help the clinician understand why a patient may behave in a certain way with regards to his or her oral health.

Question 3: How do you provide support?

There are often times in practice when patients need support. It can be easy sometimes to focus on what needs to be done and to tell someone what he or she needs to do. This has the disadvantage of taking away the patient's feelings of autonomy and increasing resistance. It can also make the patient feel as if his or her efforts to date are unnoticed. It is difficult to feel that further changes are worthwhile if the ones that have already been made are insignificant.

Affirmations that demonstrate appreciation for the patient's efforts can be useful in helping the patient believe that he or she has the ability to change.

This brings us to the second of the OARS—"affirmations." Affirmations demonstrate appreciation for the patient's efforts and reinforce positive acts. Offering short words of appreciation for the small achievements patients have made, and encouraging them to persevere, can be useful in helping the patient believe that he or she has the ability to change (Bandura 1995). Affirmations also create and maintain rapport, encouraging the patient to talk through his or her feelings about behavior change with the clinician. Affirmations can reflect on the content of what the patient has said. Some examples of this are:

"You took time to think this through ..."

"You've thought about how you might handle things ..."

"You are trying to keep up the flossing even though you find it a struggle ..."

"You've managed to cut down with your smoking over the past couple of weeks ..."

"You didn't want to come today, but you did anyway ..."

Affirmations also acknowledge the patient's positive qualities and make him or her feel noticed as a person:

"You are the kind of person who always does his or her best ..."

"You are the kind of person who tries to be responsible ..."

It is important to get the level of affirmation within a consultation right. Affirmations are useful to express appreciation for the patient and enhance rapport, but doing it too much could potentially lead the patient to believe that the clinician does not genuinely mean what he or she says. The general recommendation is to include them, but not to excess. The patient is the best indicator of whether affirmation is useful—if he or she seems uncomfortable or skeptical at any point, this should signal to the clinician that the number of affirmations he or she is making should be reduced.

Question 4: How do you convey understanding?

Asking open questions and making affirmations are excellent ways of gathering information from the patient. However, while asking questions is often a first step in eliciting important information, questions do not convey to the patient that he or she has been understood.

Moving on to the third of the OARS, another excellent way of building and maintaining rapport, by demonstrating respect, understanding, and encouraging the patient to elaborate further, is through the use of "reflective listening."

Reflective listening

It is often assumed that when we have listened to somebody else, we understand what is meant by what the person said. Listening is generally a passive process—the listener remains quiet and hears what the other person is saying. However, unless the listener checks what he or she has understood, it cannot be assumed that the listener accurately understands the other person's meaning. This is illustrated in the example below, where the clinician uses a mainly questioning approach:

> Patient: "I know I should floss, but I just never remember."
> Clinician: "Well, when do you try to do it?"
> Patient: "That's just it. I don't really have a set time and most of the time I forget altogether."
> Clinician: "What about flossing after you brush your teeth?"
> Patient: "Yes, that would be good and I try to do it, but I still never seem to remember. My life is really busy and stressful right now."
> Clinician: "Do you ever forget to brush your teeth?"
> Patient: "Yes, but not very often."

> Clinician: "So what about committing to flossing once per day after you brush?"
>
> Patient: "I guess I could try that, but it's what I've been trying to do and I really haven't been able to stick to it."
>
> Clinician: "Well, given that flossing is really important to prevent tooth decay and gum disease, you really should be doing it on a regular basis. You are going to really avoid some problems if you can get yourself on a schedule and really stick to it. I really think that you need to make a commitment. Can you do that?"
>
> Patient: "Yes, but I'm just afraid that I might not be able to do it right now.

In the example above, the clinician is adopting a mainly directing style and is not taking the time to listen to the patient. The patient is clearly saying things that indicate the clinician's suggestions have not worked in practice. There is little exploration with the patient about what he or she thinks might work. The clinician is assuming an expert role, despite the fact that the patient is the expert in what might best fit in with his or her life. The rapport between the patient and clinician is clearly damaged.

There is a clear gap between what the patient says and the clinician understanding about what the patient means. To address that gap, listening needs to be an active process. Reflective listening involves making a statement in reply to what the patient has just said in order to demonstrate understanding. Figure 3.2 shows how the process of reflective listening works (Gordon 1970).

> Reflective listening enables the listener to check what he or she has understood from what the speaker has said. Moreover, it enables the speaker to feel understood.

Reflective listening serves two functions. Firstly, it enables the listener to check what he or she has understood from what the speaker has said. Secondly, it enables the speaker to feel understood (in turn enhancing the rapport between the two parties), and it also encourages the speaker to elaborate and give more detail. This again is useful for the clinician. By using reflective listening when talking about behavior change, a lot of clinically relevant information can be sought from the patient, while at the same time promoting a good rapport and an atmosphere of understanding. It also takes the pressure off the clinician, giving him or her the space to develop a curious mindset and to really understand what is being said, rather than being forced to try to guess what the patient's issues might be all the time.

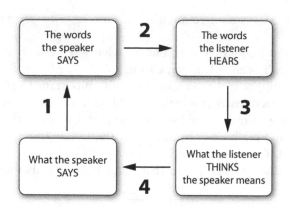

Figure 3.2. Reflective listening.

There are two broad types of reflections that can be made: *Content reflections* are short summaries of what the patient has just said, whereas *meaning reflections* are deeper and focus on the meaning implied by what the patient has just said. For example, if a patient said:

> "I should probably try to avoid the sweets—my teeth are in a terrible state."

a content reflection of this might be:

> "You see a connection between what you eat and developing cavities."

whereas, a meaning reflection would be:

> "You want to try to avoid having more fillings in the future."

Forming reflections can be difficult at first. One good way to think about forming reflective listening statements is to think, "It sounds like … ," which enables the clinician to practice making a reflection of what he or she has understood. Some clinicians may choose to include the "it sounds like" in their reflection, but as skill increases, this can be dropped from the reflection, leaving simply the statement of what has been understood.

It is important to note at this point that in reflective listening, the clinician is making a statement. For this reason, when making a reflection, it is essential to remember to make the intonation go *down* at the end of the statement.

Allowing the intonation to go up would turn a reflection into a question, suggesting inquisition rather than understanding. This could result in an interaction similar to the one in the example above.

At first, this form of "verbal listening" can feel strange—when a person is responding to show that he or she is listening, it is usually done or achieved through non-verbal cues. If a person wants more information, it is a natural reaction to want to ask a question. It takes practice to get used to forming reflective listening statements, but it pays off within the consultation in terms of developing good rapport and employing a guiding style of communication. This is illustrated in the following example:

Patient: "I know I should floss, but I just never remember."

Clinician: "You know that it's important, but you often forget."

Patient: "Yeah, I know that I should be doing it, I just don't."

Clinician: "So even though you know it's important, something is getting in the way of your doing it."

Patient: "Yes, I always seem to be in too much of a rush, and then when I could do it, I might forget ... I guess in the big scheme of things, I'm not sure if it's as important as other things I need to do and sometimes I just can't get it all done."

Clinician: "So you have a hard time remembering and making time for it because you're not really sure if flossing is as important as other things that have to get done."

Patient: "Yes, but I really don't want to end up like my parents. They had terrible gum disease and lost most of their teeth. I just don't want that to happen."

Clinician: "So you want to find a solution so you don't end up in the same position as your parents."

Patient: "Yes, I really don't want that."

Clinician: "It's important to you to take care of your teeth so that you don't one day find you lose them."

Patient: "Yes. I have had a really hard time flossing in the morning or at night when I brush because I'm always in a hurry to go to work or get to bed. I suppose I should just make it more of a priority, and doing it right before bed wouldn't be that hard, but the mornings are impossible ... It would be great if I could make it more convenient."

Clinician: "So, although not ideal, you could probably pull it off at night. But you definitely need to find a time other than first thing in the morning."

Patient: "Well actually, I'm thinking that I always like to zone out in front of the TV for an hour or so before getting ready for bed. If I had the floss handy it would probably be quite easy to floss while I watch TV."

Clinician: "Flossing while you're watching TV could work."

Patient: "Yes, actually I think it would."

Clinician: "What do you think about giving that a try?"

Patient: "Yeah, I'm going to try that. I think I'll keep the floss next to my remote control so that I get reminded to floss every time I sit down and watch TV. I know I won't forget to watch TV, so this should help."

We can see in the example above that the clinician takes time to understand the patient through reflective listening and helps the patient to suggest his own solution to the problem. By not providing answers, or continually asking questions about the things the clinician thinks the patient should do, this gives the patient the opportunity to explore how he feels about flossing and allows him to remain in control.

Reflective listening is a useful skill that

• makes the patient feel understood,

• encourages the patient to clarify what he or she means,

• gives the clinician space to process meaningful clinical information,

• develops and maintains good rapport,

• enables patients to explore their current behavior, how they would like to be, and how they feel about making changes, and

• helps the clinician to understand the patient's perspective on health behavior change.

Question 5: How do you get information across?

A common reaction on the part of clinicians to patients employing damaging health behaviors is to put them back on the right track by telling them what they should do and why they should do it (commonly known as the "righting reflex"). There is a general belief held within health care contexts, upon which much policy and training is based, that providing information leads to a change in the patient's attitude, which in turn leads to changes in behavior (Morrison and Bennett 2006).

When used in this fashion, information is rarely reduced to its bare facts and is often combined with the clinician's interpretation of its relevance for the person. However, as we saw in chapter 2, and by reflecting on our own clinical experiences, where patients are given information in the hope that this will trigger change, such practice is often ineffective. This is because without encouraging the patient to actively assess the relevance of the information to his or her own situation, it does not lead the patient to draw personal meaning from it. This makes the information easier to discount or ignore. It has been suggested, therefore, that the more information is evaluated and applied by the recipient of it, the more likely it is that such information will be taken on board (Wilding and Valentine 1997).

Another issue is that of redundant information. To what extent is the patient already aware of what the clinician is telling him or her? One challenge in clinical practice commonly raised by health professionals is the lack of time they have to spend with each patient. Time is precious; thus, telling the patient things that they already know is a waste of that time.

Within the style of guiding, however, there are of course times when information needs to be conveyed to the patient. At these times, it is important for clinicians to ask themselves whether they are addressing a genuine requirement for information or whether they are feeling that righting reflex and hoping that providing information will change the patient's current behavior.

What is clear is that in order to be effective, information needs to add to the patient's existing knowledge, and it needs to be seen as personally relevant by the patient. One way in which the clinician can seek to achieve this is through the elicit-provide-elicit method.

Step 1: Assess what the patient already knows

Examples to assess the patient's knowledge include:

> "What do you already know about ...?"

> "How much do you know about ...?"

COMMUNICATION AND HEALTH
BEHAVIOR CHANGE COUNSELLING

> "It sounds like you already know quite a lot about ... Tell me what else you know."

Step 2: Provide further information

Always ask permission before giving information, to maintain a good rapport. Keep information to the bare facts, rather than interpreting it on behalf of the patient.

Examples on how to stick to the facts include:

> "Some patients find that ..."

> "Research has shown that ..."

> "One thing that improves this condition is ..."

Step 3: Elicit what the information means for the patient

Check what the patient understands from the information given and its personal relevance.

Examples on how to elicit from the patient include:

> "What do you think about that information?"

> "What does that mean for you?"

> "What do you understand from that?"

Exchanging information is a useful skill to employ in clinical practice because

- it enables the patient to add to his or her existing knowledge,

- it encourages the patient to actively evaluate the information and draw personal meaning from it,

• it saves the clinician time, and

• it maintains good rapport.

This approach to *exchanging,* rather than *giving* information, aims to primarily assess what the patient already knows about the topic, then to contribute to that existing understanding, and finally to establish what the patient sees as personal implications from that information.

Question 6: How do you bring it all together?

Before moving on in the dental visit it is important to summarize and demonstrate to the patient that the clinician has listened, understood, and taken on board what the patient has said.

There are times during the consultation when it is appropriate to move on. Before doing so, it is important to demonstrate to the patient that the clinician has listened, understood, and taken on board what the patient has said. This can be achieved through the fourth of the OARS skills, "summarizing" what the patient has said. Summaries are similar to reflections but are lengthier. They can be used to bring together all the things the patient has said regarding a particular clinical issue, to link some things a patient has said with other things he or she has said at another point in the session, or to bring a discussion to a close. Summaries are also useful tools for the clinician to consider what the patient has said and to consider how the patient feels about making particular changes.

A collecting summary *(brings together key issues raised by the patient)*:

> "So, you've been finding that your gums have been bleeding when you brush your teeth for some time. Until you saw a recent advertisement about gum disease, you thought this was pretty normal, but now you've started to feel a little worried. You have tried different mouthwashes that you think might have helped and have seen no difference. You don't know what else you can do, and hope I might be able to help you with this."

A linking summary *(links together what the patient has said about the topic)*:

> "So giving up smoking is a big challenge for you. On the one hand, you really enjoy it. It's part of your social life, part of who you are. It helps you to take time out and gives you space to relax. Every time you've tried to give up before, you've been clawing the wall—giving it up is hard, and it's as much about how smoking makes you feel rather than just withdrawal from the nicotine. On the other hand, you know smoking is bad for you, and you think it has probably contributed to your gum problems. It costs a lot. It smells. You said you would like to give it up but don't know if you could."

A wrapping-up summary *(to close a session, or move the discussion on)*:

> "OK, so just to summarize, you've talked a bit about what you eat in a typical day. You eat quite a lot of healthy food—you always eat vegetables with a meal. You feel that you eat quite a lot of convenience foods that are high in sugar. You know that it's not good for your teeth, but it's often much quicker and easier because you lead quite a busy life. The family like sugary foods too, which again makes it hard to change what you eat. You've said that you would like to make changes to your diet because you want to reduce your risk of further cavities, and you'd also like to lose a bit of weight. You've tried cutting these foods out before. In the long term it didn't work so you're not confident you would succeed if you tried again. Does that sound right to you?"

Summarizing is useful in

- demonstrating that the clinician has understood the essence of what the patient has said overall,

- showing that what the patient has said has been taken on board,

- maintaining cohesiveness and rapport,

- highlighting that the patient feels different ways about changing his or her health behavior, and

- double checking that no important issues have been forgotten.

SUMMARY

When talking about health behavior change with patients, it is important to be sensitive to how they might feel about change. Some patients may feel ready to start making changes. Others may have more pressing issues that require addressing and need to be followed to clarify this. For patients who are ambivalent about making changes, a guiding style may be most appropriate.

Using the basic communication skills of Open questions, Affirmations, Reflections, and Summaries (OARS), and exchanging rather than simply giving information, can help the clinician to employ a guiding style with patients who are struggling to change. This is summarized in Table 3.1.

Enabling patients to feel understood and encouraged to take an active role in how and why to change their health behavior can encourage them to constructively discuss their own reasons for and against change, rather than simply becoming resistant in the consultation.

These skills are the foundation for helping patients to increase their motivation to make changes. Chapter 6 will present how using these skills in a refined way during Motivational Interviewing can help patients resolve their

Table 3.1. Summary of OARS.

Skill	Description	Example
Open question	A way of eliciting greater patient response to a request for information	"How do you feel about ..."
Affirmation	A way to build patient confidence and enhance rapport by recognizing the positives	"You can see you did really well ..."
Reflective listening	A way to express understanding and validate the patient while facilitating increased discussion and patient engagement	"It sounds like you ..."
Summarizing	An empathic way to sum up, link different parts of the conversation, or wrap up	"So let me see if I have this right, so far you have said that ..."
Exchanging information	A way to find out what the patient already knows and to increase their knowledge in a way that actively engages them in the process	"What do you know about ..."

COMMUNICATION AND HEALTH BEHAVIOR CHANGE COUNSELLING

ambivalence to change their health behavior. There are also a number of brief intervention tools that can help the clinician alongside these basic communication skills, which are discussed in chapter 5.

ACKNOWLEDGMENTS

Thanks to Judith Carpenter for the reflective listening diagram and to Delwyn Catley for the clinical examples of a questioning versus a reflective listening approach and the OARS summary table.

REFERENCES

Bandura, A.E. (ed.). (1995). *Self-Efficacy in Changing Societies*. New York: Cambridge University Press.

Brehm, J.W. (1966). *A Theory of Psychological Reactance*. New York: Academic Press.

Department of Health. (2004). *Choosing Health: Making Healthy Choices Easier*. Norwich, England: Department of Health.

Gordon, T. (ed.). (1970). *PET: Parent Effectiveness Training*. New York: Wyden.

Morrison, V., and P. Bennett (eds.). (2006). *An Introduction to Health Psychology*. Upper Saddle River, NJ: Pearson/Prentice Hall.

Najavits, L.M., P. Crits-Christoph, et al. (2000). Clinicians' impact on the quality of substance use disorder treatment. *Subst Use Misuse* 35(12–14):2161–2190.

Rollnick, S., P. Mason, et al. (eds.). (1999). *Health Behaviour Change: A Guide for Practitioners*. Edinburgh: Harcourt Brace.

Rollnick, S., W.R. Miller, et al. (eds.). (2007). *Motivational Interviewing in Health Care*. New York: Guilford Press.

Wilding, J., and E. Valentine (eds.). (1997). *Superior Memory*. London: Psychology Press.

CHAPTER 4

MOTIVATIONAL INTERVIEWING (MI) AND ITS BASIC TOOLS

Delwyn Catley, Kathy Goggin, and Ian Lynam

Key Points of This Chapter

- Motivational Interviewing offers both a style and particular methods or techniques that can be incorporated into counselling interactions to increase the likelihood of patient behavior change.
- Motivational Interviewing is based on the assumption that individuals are motivated to change when change is connected to something *they* value.
- The MI method places great importance on the nature of the relationship between the clinician and the patient.
- In MI, developing discrepancy involves exploring with patients the gap between their goals or values, or how they ideally would like things to be, and their current behavior.
- The means for facilitating change is based on developing discrepancy and exploring the assumed ambivalence felt by patients regarding change.
- The spirit of MI consists of three major elements: collaboration (clinicians foster a partnership with their patients), evocation (clinicians emphasize eliciting the motivation from "within" their patients), and autonomy (clinicians allow freedom of their patients to make their own choices).
- In implementing MI, the following major principles are being followed: express empathy (by communicating acceptance and using reflective listening), develop discrepancy (by exploring the patients' current behavior and their important goals or values), roll with resistance (by avoiding arguing with the patients), and support self-efficacy (by seeking to increase the patients' optimism and confidence that they can change).
- In MI, the four main communication skills can be used as summarized by the acronym OARS, which stands for "open questions," "affirmations," "reflective listening," and "summarizing."

INTRODUCTION

As an exercise to get started, we ask how important you think it is to use Motivational Interviewing with your patients. Please select a number from the scale below:

0 1 2 3 4 5 6 7 8 9 10

No importance   Extreme importance

We have used this importance ruler at the beginning of Motivational Interviewing trainings for the past several years. If your score follows the typical pattern of responses we have observed, the score would fall within a range of 3 to 8. Even among audiences that have freely chosen to take valuable time to attend our workshops, we find that most do not rate the importance of using MI as a 10. We believe that this reflects some ambivalence among participants regarding the use of MI. If this is how you answered, it is a perfect position to be in, as this chapter discusses further elements of behavior change. In Motivational Interviewing, ambivalence is viewed as typical for people who are considering a behavior change. Rather than seeing patients as resistant, the assumption in MI is that it is normal for patients to be ambivalent, therefore representing an opportunity. An opportunity exists because ambivalence, by definition, indicates that while a person may have some hesitation about change, he or she also has some interest in change.

WHAT IS MOTIVATIONAL INTERVIEWING?

"Motivational Interviewing is a method of communication rather than a set of techniques. It is not a bag of tricks for getting people to do what they don't want to do. It is not something that one does to people; rather, it is a fundamental way of being with and for people—a facilitative approach to communication that evokes natural change" (Miller and Rollnick 2002).

MI is a style or method of counselling patients that initially grew out of work to help individuals with addictions. One of the founders of the method, William Miller, had observed that whereas counsellors often favored confrontational methods of counselling, research findings pointed toward the benefit of a non-confrontational approach characterized by a strong alliance or bond between counsellor and patient (Miller 1983). Miller began to develop an empathy-based approach with a focus on the perspective of the patient in understanding the challenge of behavior change. Together with the work of Stephen Rollnick, who had been focusing on patients' ambivalence regarding change, they co-founded the development of MI (Miller and Rollnick 1991, 2002). While MI was initially most commonly associated with addiction treatment and more traditional counselling settings, it has become apparent that MI can be exceedingly useful in a wide variety of healthcare settings (Resnicow et al. 2002). For example, patients seen in dental settings are often counselled regarding oral hygiene, dietary habits, and smoking cessation. Patient engagement and adherence to clinician recommendations are also central to effective dental treatment outcomes. MI offers both a style and particular methods or techniques that can be incorporated into counselling interactions to help increase the likelihood of patient behavior change. In the sections that follow, we briefly review the research evidence for MI, particularly as it relates to counselling patients in dental settings, and then provide an overview of the underpinnings and methods of MI. For those who would like to study more, we highly recommend Miller and Rollnick's lucid and readable book, which expands considerably on the information provided here (Miller and Rollnick 2002).

> Motivational Interviewing offers both a style and particular methods or techniques that can be incorporated into counselling interactions to increase the likelihood of patient behavior change.

Research evidence for MI

The efficacy of MI has been examined in numerous studies across a wide array of behavior change domains. To date, there have been four published meta-analyses summarizing the literature (Burke et al. 2003, 2004; Hettema et al. 2005; Rubak et al. 2005) providing support for the efficacy of MI. The meta-analyses indicate that MI-based interventions are at least as effective as other active treatments and superior to no-treatment or placebo controls for a range of problems involving addictive behavior (drugs, alcohol, and gambling), diet and exercise, treatment engagement, retention, and adherence. Importantly, the reviews indicate that MI is highly efficient compared to other methods (Burke et al. 2004), with as little as 15 minutes of interaction shown to be effective in the majority of studies (Rubak et al. 2005). Furthermore, effectiveness does not appear to depend on MI being delivered by counselling experts. Rubak and co-workers found a significant effect in 80% of studies where MI was delivered by physicians (Rubak et al. 2005).

Of particular relevance to dental settings are studies of dietary habits, smoking, and oral hygiene. As the aforementioned meta-analyses indicate, MI is effective for addressing changes in dietary habits including changes in overall dietary intake (Mhurchu et al. 1998), fat intake (Bowen et al. 2002; Mhurchu et al. 1998), carbohydrate consumption (Mhurchu et al. 1998), and consumption of fruits and vegetables (Resnicow et al. 2001; Richards et al. 2006). Evidence from smoking cessation literature is less strong, with meta-analyses not finding support for MI, partially limited by a lack of studies. However, there is evidence that MI leads to more attempts to quit (Borrelli et al. 2005; Wakefield et al. 2004), reductions in smoking level (Borrelli et al. 2005), and increased readiness to quit (Butler et al. 1999). Significant effects on smoking cessation, though less commonly observed, have been reported in some studies (Curry 2003; Pbert et al. 2006; Soria et al. 2006; Valanis et al. 2001). Given that there is currently no established alternative for motivating smokers to quit in clinical settings, MI represents a promising avenue toward progress.

Studies of MI for oral hygiene have been limited to date. Weinstein and co-workers compared MI to traditional health education among a sample of 240 mothers of young children with high risk for developing dental caries (Weinstein et al. 2004, 2006). The focus was on the use of dietary and non-dietary behaviors for caries prevention and compared an MI session, six follow-up calls, a pamphlet, and a video to the pamphlet and video alone. The addition of the single MI session and follow-up calls led to significantly fewer new dental caries among the children after 2 years.

In a recent study by Almomani and co-workers, it was found that the use of MI in a controlled clinical trial was able to significantly improve oral hygiene status over a period of 8 weeks in individuals with severe mental illness (Almomani et al. 2009). Additional benefits from an MI-based counselling approach on oral hygiene status were reported in a two patient case-series study by Jönsson and co-workers (2009). In both patients, a significant improvement of oral hygiene and gingival inflammation status was achieved and maintained over an observation period of 2 years (Jönsson et al. 2009).

What triggers behavior change?

While the research support for the efficacy of MI is strong, at this point less is known about how and why MI works. Nevertheless, MI was developed with a particular understanding of how behavior change occurs. Traditional approaches to counselling patients in settings such as dental practices tend to focus on educating patients. The implicit assumption is that increased patient knowledge (e.g., the role of plaque in dental diseases or the harmful effects of smoking) will translate into behavior change. As this is rarely the case, an educational approach alone often leads to clinician and patient frustration, poor outcomes, and a sense of futility in counselling.

MI is based on the assumption that individuals are motivated to change when change is connected to something *they* value. This is distinct from "external" reasons for changing provided by a clinician, such as:

"You should quit smoking because it will prevent gum disease."

The MI approach instead begins with an exploration of *the patient's* view of the potential benefits of changing by saying:

"Tell me about any benefits you see in quitting smoking."

As indicated in our opening exercise, it is also assumed that in the vast majority of cases, patients are ambivalent about change. The key point about ambivalence is that it implies individuals have both reasons to change and reasons not to change. All too often conversations become bogged down by an exclusive focus on all the reasons individuals don't want to change. Clinicians are often drawn into a form of discussion where they are arguing for change or trying to persuade the patient, while the patient argues against change by providing obstacles and barriers. The goal of MI is to avoid this pitfall by the willingness to explore *both* sides of a patient's ambivalence to help him or her consider what he or she truly values.

> Motivational Interviewing is based on the assumption that individuals are motivated to change when change is connected to something *they* value.

Motivation and the clinician-patient relationship

As mentioned in chapter 3, the MI method also places great importance on the nature of the relationship between the clinician and the patient. This relationship is often enhanced when fostered in an environment of mutual respect, while acknowledging the common thread of humanity that links the clinician and the patient. Whereas clinicians are often cast in the "expert role,"

> The MI method places great importance on the nature of the relationship between the clinician and the patient.

the strength of the bond between clinician and patient can often be enhanced when the clinician recognizes the "expertise" of the patient regarding his or her own life. Clinicians may be more effective when they see themselves as needing to learn from the patient the opportunities for improving patient health. Viewing the relationship from this perspective encourages a mutual partnership. The patient and clinician work toward a common goal in a manner that makes the patient feel supported. Training in MI often encourages clinicians to experience the receiving end of counselling for a behavior change about which they feel ambivalent. Heightened awareness of what it is like to be a patient encourages greater empathy and the appreciation of the importance of clinician support. In the "'Spirit' of MI" section below, we elaborate further on elements considered essential for creating a relationship between clinician and patient that is effective in facilitating behavior change.

> In MI, developing discrepancy involves exploring with patients the gap between their goals or values, or how they ideally would like things to be, and their current behavior.

MI also focuses particular attention on ways the clinician's actions can foster or undermine patient motivation. Unfortunately, it is quite easy to undermine motivation despite very good intentions. As mentioned in chapter 3, Miller and Rollnick have coined the term "righting reflex" (the urge to "try to put things right") to describe the tendency that counsellors have to lecture or persuade patients of the wisdom of making a particular change (Miller and Rollnick 2002). Often this approach leads patients to feel pressured and to, paradoxically, resist change. MI aims to avoid lecturing or persuading. Instead, the goal is to focus on *developing discrepancy*. Developing discrepancy involves exploring with patients the gap between their goals or values, or how they ideally would like things to be, and their current behavior. For example, research indicates that most people who are smokers actually would prefer to be non-smokers (Centers for Disease Control and Prevention 2002). While this aspiration does not necessarily translate into the desire to quit *today*, it does highlight that there is an underlying source of motivation to be tapped. In the vast majority of cases, individuals do ideally want to live in a healthy manner, leaving room for a discussion of that goal and how they could move closer to it.

During this process, the clinician also attempts to *elicit* "change talk" or statements that are consistent with or in the direction of making a change, for example by hearing the patient say:

"Even though I'm not really doing it, I would like to be eating healthier."

In the earliest stages of considering a change, so-called change talk often takes the form of simply recognizing or acknowledging there is a problem, again, for example, by hearing the patient say:

"I know I should brush more regularly."

In the later stages this often takes the form of expressing optimism or the intention to change and, therefore, the patient may say:

"I'll definitely start brushing and flossing twice a day."

The key issue is that the clinician has the ability to influence the relationship between clinician and patient to either foster resistance or develop discrepancy and elicit change talk.

Giving advice is something that most of us are very familiar with. However, unsolicited advice is generally not very pleasant to receive. This is perhaps even truer when it comes to unsolicited advice about our behavior or health practices (e.g., quitting smoking, losing weight, adhering to medications). Take the following example:

Patient: "I feel like my teeth are really stained, is there anything I can do?"
Clinician: "Yes, you really need to quit smoking."
Patient: "Yes, but it's not that easy."
Clinician: "No, it's not easy, but you need to do it and not just for the sake of your teeth but also for your overall health."
Patient: "Yes, I know I should quit but it's just not that easy for me. Isn't there something else you can do?"
Clinician: "Not really ... Have you tried to quit using nicotine gum or patch?"
Patient: "Yes, I've considered it, but that stuff's really expensive and I'm not sure it will work for me."
Clinician: "It will work if you are committed. I think the real key is for you to be fully committed to quitting."
Patient: "I suppose, but with all I've got going I'm just not committed right now ... So there's nothing else that can be done?"

This excerpt highlights the common dynamic of a clinician arguing for change, while the patient makes "yes, but" counterarguments. If the clinician's goal is to help the patient make a change, a different approach might be warranted.

Definition of MI

> The means for facilitating change is based on developing discrepancy and exploring the assumed ambivalence felt by patients regarding change.

At this point, it is useful to consider a formal definition of MI. Rollnick and Miller have defined MI as "a client-centred, directive method for enhancing intrinsic motivation to change by exploring and resolving ambivalence" (Rollnick and Miller 1995). MI is client or patient-centered in that the clinician attempts to work from the patient's perspective. As we have discussed, rather than the clinician providing his or her reasons for recommending a particular health behavior, the clinician attempts to elicit from the patient whatever reasons *he or she* has for engaging in that health behavior. Research evidence indicates that these intrinsic or "internal" reasons for change tend to be associated with greater adherence to medical recommendations, persistence, and long-term behavior change (Ryan and Deci 2000).

Although the approach is patient-centred, the clinician is nonetheless directive in that there is the goal of exploring and attempting to facilitate change in a particular direction (e.g., to brush twice daily, to floss more frequently, to avoid sugary foods, etc.). The means for facilitating that change is based on developing discrepancy and exploring the assumed ambivalence felt by patients regarding change. As an MI(-minded) clinician, therefore, you take specific steps to explore ambivalence and facilitate the patient's resolution of ambivalence in the direction of making a healthy change.

"SPIRIT" OF MI

Miller and Rollnick have emphasized that in practicing MI it is more important to embody the "spirit" or philosophy of MI than to employ specific techniques (Miller and Rollnick 2002). The methods and techniques of MI are useful, but only insofar as they are conducted in a manner consistent with the underlying philosophy.

The spirit of MI consists of three major elements: *collaboration, evocation,* and *autonomy.* Collaboration refers to a style of working *with* the patient. In the MI method, the clinician fosters a partnership with the patient rather than assuming an expert role in which the patient is a recipient. The clinician and the patient work together toward a common goal as the clinician actively seeks to diminish his or her expert role.

The element of evocation refers to a style that emphasizes eliciting the motivation from "within" the patient rather than trying to impose motivation from the "outside." Rather than making arguments for change, the clinician will guide the *patient* to examine and resolve his or her ambivalence. The style is also calm and eliciting, with no need for the clinician to use high-energy, high-pressure, or confrontational tactics to bring about change.

> The spirit of MI consists of three major elements: collaboration (clinicians foster a partnership with their patients), evocation (clinicians emphasize eliciting the motivation from "within" their patients), and autonomy (clinicians allow freedom of their patients to make their own choices).

The evocative style is facilitated by the third element of the spirit: patient autonomy. MI emphasizes the freedom of patients to make their own choices. The responsibility for change is not in the hands of the clinician. Rather the role of the clinician is to facilitate a productive exploration of the possibility of change. At the end of the day, the final decision on what to do rests with the patient. Paradoxically, the more clinicians emphasize patients' autonomy, the greater their internal motivation to change is likely to be (Ryan and Deci 2000; Williams et al. 2000).

The implementation of these elements often leads clinicians to report that counselling is more enjoyable, less effortful, and more productive. They often feel a burden is lifted when they allow patients to have autonomy and they do not have to be the expert on how to solve the patient's problems or feel responsible for the patient's ultimate decision. The result is in the sense of working with the patient rather than pushing for change (see Figure 4.1).

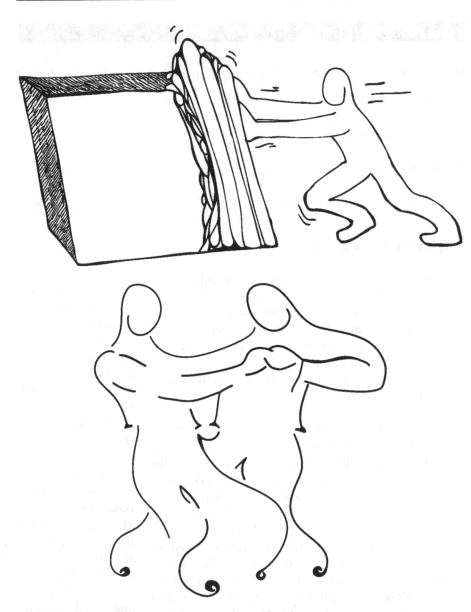

Figure 4.1. Spirit of MI. Artwork by J. Brendan O'Shaughnessy.

MAJOR PRINCIPLES

In implementing the spirit of MI there are four major principles:

• express empathy,

• develop discrepancy,

• roll with resistance, and

• support self-efficacy and optimism.

Express empathy

The first principle, to *express empathy*, highlights the importance of the patient's perspective. The term "empathy" refers to understanding the perspective of another person. In MI, it is not sufficient to *have* empathy; rather it is important to demonstrate that understanding by *expressing* it. This is achieved when communicating acceptance and using reflective listening skills.

Communicating acceptance or avoiding judgment, no matter how much it conflicts with one's individual convictions, is essential for developing true empathy and fostering the collaboration that is central to MI. Patients who feel judged or criticized will be very unlikely to engage in a meaningful conversation about change. Rather, patients will be more likely to engage if their perspective is acknowledged or validated by the clinician. Viewed from the outside, a patient's behavior may seem inexplicable or wrong-headed. However, when understood in the context of the patient's particular view of the situation, the behavior usually makes a lot more sense. When a clinician communicates understanding to a patient, the perspective is not unreasonable or judged negatively, therefore the patient's urge to self-defend is *reduced*. This increases the likelihood that the patient will be able to focus on a more productive agenda—the consideration of alternative perspectives and options, and the possibility of change.

> In implementing MI, the following major principles are being followed: express empathy (by communicating acceptance and using reflective listening), develop discrepancy (by exploring patients' current behavior and their important goals or values), roll with resistance (by avoiding arguing with the patients), and support self-efficacy (by seeking to increase patients' optimism and confidence that they can change).

Develop discrepancy

The second major principle is to *develop discrepancy* between the patient's current behavior and his or her important goals or values. For example, a patient may have a goal of being a good parent. Eating in a healthy way and modelling good oral hygiene practices may be an important way to live out the value of being a good parent. As noted, most patients want to be healthy and have that as a goal. Discrepancy and, therefore, motivation can be developed by exploring how current behavior fits in or could be changed to achieve that goal.

Roll with resistance

The third general principle is that the clinician *rolls with resistance* and avoids arguing. Rolling with resistance involves the use of specific methods for responding to resistance that avoid "pushing back." Pushing back, persuading, or arguing tends to increase resistance, so the MI clinician instead attempts to roll with resistance to deflect or minimize it.

Support self-efficacy

The fourth principle is to *support self-efficacy* (or confidence) and optimism for change. A wealth of research (Bandura 1997) indicates that individuals who have confidence in their abilities to engage in a particular behavior are much more likely to engage in that behavior. A clinician who communicates doubt regarding the ability or likelihood of a patient to succeed with making a change will undermine the patient's self-efficacy. MI clinicians therefore seek to increase their patients' optimism and confidence that they can change.

OARS: BASIC TOOLS FOR BUILDING MOTIVATION TO CHANGE

In MI, the four main communication skills can be used as summarized by the acronym OARS, which stands for "open questions," "affirmations," "reflective listening," and "summarizing."

As introduced in chapter 2, the basic tools for building motivation to change can be summarized with the acronym **OARS**:

- Open questions,

- Affirmations,

- Reflective listening, and

- Summarizing.

MOTIVATIONAL INTERVIEWING (MI) AND ITS BASIC TOOLS

Use open-ended questions

In contrast to closed questions, open questions are those that cannot be answered with a simple "yes" or "no" or other one-word answer. Open questions lead the patient to talk more, providing more of a picture of the situation as he or she sees it. This aids the clinician in developing empathy (i.e., to understand the patient's perspective) and reduces the clinician's burden by increasing the likelihood that the *patient* is doing the talking and thinking. A general rule when using open questions is to avoid asking three or more questions consecutively.

Examples of open questions are:

> "I'd like to learn a little bit more about the routine for taking care of your teeth. How do you go about cleaning your teeth?"

> "Tell me about your smoking."

> "To what extent ..."

> "Help me understand ..."

Affirm patients

The second basic tool is affirming. Affirming patients can enhance rapport and help support patients' confidence. Affirmations aim to recognize patients' strengths:

> "You are a very determined person ..."

> "It's clear that it is important to you to be a good spouse ..."

and efforts:

> "You've really tried to work on this ..."

"You've already made some efforts to be healthier ..."

Affirmations should be specific and genuine, rather than general overenthusiastic statements. Other examples include:

"That's a wonderful idea."

"Thanks for being willing to discuss this."

"I've really enjoyed getting to know more about you."

Use reflective listening

The third basic MI tool is reflective listening. Reflective listening is a method of responding to a patient in which the clinician repeats or paraphrases what he or she has heard the patient say. Two examples of reflective statements are given below. In the first example, as mentioned in chapter 3, the reflection may begin with:

"It sounds like ..."

This is a useful way to learn to make reflections because it helps to ensure what follows will be a reflection of what the clinician understood the patient to say. When reflecting becomes more automatic, the "It sounds like ..." part can simply be dropped. Other examples:

Patient: "A lot of the time everything just becomes too much and I need a cigarette."
Clinician: "It sounds like you often smoke because you feel overwhelmed."
Patient: "Well, I floss off and on I suppose"
Clinician: "Your flossing is not that regular."

The purpose of reflective listening is to affirm and validate the patient's perspective. It communicates acceptance and empathy by demonstrating to the patient that he or she is being listened to and that his or her perspective is understood.

It also serves to keep the patient thinking and talking. This is because it is typical for the patient to respond to a reflective statement with *elaboration*. For example, in response to a clinician who says:

> "So it sounds like you find it hard to resist candy."

a patient might answer:

> "Yes, that's right. If I have it around I just can't keep my hand out of the jar ... I guess I should work on keeping it out of the house if I ever want to stop!"

Without the clinician needing to use frequent or insightful questioning, the patient reveals more about his or her perspective on the problem.

But what if the clinician is inaccurate in the reflection? Typically a patient will simply correct the clinician:

> "Well, no, that's not quite right, I do try to floss regularly but I find that ..."

One other aspect of reflective listening that is useful to keep in mind is that reflections can be made at varying levels of "depth." Reflecting the essential meaning or inferring the essence of what a patient is saying demonstrates most powerfully to the patient that the clinician is truly "getting" what the patient is saying. For example, to a patient who says:

> "I keep trying and trying to quit smoking, but I always end up relapsing, and then I have to face my family again ..."

a clinician might at a surface level say:

> "You've tried to quit many times but you've always gone back to smoking, and that makes it hard for you to face your family."

A clinician making a deeper reflection, responding to meaning, might say:

> "So you very much want to be quit but you feel like you are letting your family down every time you try and fail."

Often patients will make statements that suggest they might have particular feelings. If the clinician can accurately reflect the emotion, it provides another indication of his or her high level of empathy. In the example above, an alternate reflection that focuses on feelings might be:

"You feel ashamed when you try to quit but then fail."

The feeling of shame or embarrassment was implied by the patient but not explicitly stated. Of course it is not necessary for all reflections to be "deep" reflections. However, an occasional deep reflection can go a long way in developing a strong bond with a patient and encouraging greater elaboration of the patient's perspective.

Use summaries

The fourth basic skill, summarizing, is used throughout and at the end of an MI session. The goal of summarizing is to sum up discussion in a few short sentences. This can be done to make sure that the clinician is accurately grasping the patient's perspective, to link information that has been presented that shows discrepancy (i.e., between the way the patient would ideally like things to be and current behavior), or to wrap up a session as a summary paragraph might bring closure to an article.

ELICIT CHANGE TALK

While the basic tools of MI together with appropriate communication skills (see chapter 3) are essential for developing an empathetic discussion, use of these tools does not necessarily lead to greater motivation for change. These tools may be used in a manner that deliberately attempts to foster the patient's expression of interest in making a change. In other words, while the assumption is that patients are likely to be unsure about change, the clinician actively attempts to facilitate discussion of that side of the ambivalence that is related to making a change.

Statements made by a patient that are "in the direction of change" are termed "change talk." In the earliest phases of the change process this might take the form of simply recognizing that there is a problem or that there are *disadvantages of the status quo,* for example, by saying:

"I know the fact that I'm not flossing is contributing to my gum problems."

Later in the process, change talk can take the form of recognizing the *advantages of making a change,* by saying:

> "Well it sure would be nice if I didn't have to come for hygiene appointments so often."

Eventually, a patient might express *optimism regarding making a change,* by saying:

> "I really think if I stuck with it for a while it could become part of my routine."

And finally, a patient might express *a commitment to change,* by saying:

> "I'm definitely going to floss twice a day from now on."

Recent research has suggested other ways of categorizing change talk and has emphasized the importance of patient statements of commitment to change (Amrhein et al. 2003). The overall conclusion of this study was that patient change talk within a session is important because it is predictive of subsequent behavioral outcomes. So, how exactly does one facilitate change talk? Various methods are available and are discussed below.

Evocative questions

One simple method is to use "evocative" open-ended questions. As can be seen in Table 4.1, they can be used to elicit each of the types of change talk described above. In each case, the patient's answer to the question will, by definition, be change talk.

Decisional balance or pros and cons matrix

Another method of eliciting change talk is the decisional balance or, as we usually refer to it, the pros and cons matrix (Table 4.2). With the matrix in mind (or on paper), a clinician can lead discussion through each of the elements of ambivalence felt by a patient. "Cons" of not changing and "pros"

Table 4.1. Evocative questions for each type of "change talk."

Disadvantages of the status quo	"What worries you the most about your current situation?" "What do you think will happen if you don't change anything?"
Advantages of change	"How would you like things to be different?" "What would be the advantages of making a change?"
Optimism for change	"What success have you had in the past?" "Is there anything that gives you some confidence that you could change this?"
Intention to change	"What's going to have to change for you to be completely committed?" "What would you be willing to try?"

Table 4.2. Pros and cons matrix.

	Pros	Cons
If I don't change	1	2
If I do change	4	3

of making a change will, by definition, constitute change talk. The matrix can also be simplified into just two boxes that focus on the pros and cons of changing. For example, a clinician using the matrix might begin by saying:

> "Tell me a little about what you like about or see as the pros of continuing as you are." (Box 1 of the matrix)

and then follow up, to elicit change talk, with:

> "Now, tell me a little bit about any advantages you see in making some changes." (Box 4)

In our clinical experience, it is wise to begin with the pros of not changing (Box 1), because this provides an opportunity to express empathy with the patient's perspective on his or her current behavior, before exploring the possibility of changing things. Similarly, we have also found that starting with the status quo and then ending with the advantages of changing can achieve some momentum for change. For the same reasons, if using the full four-box matrix, we recommend following the boxes in the numerical order in which they are labelled.

The importance ruler

Assessing a patient's motivation for making a change can also be an opportunity for eliciting change talk. The "importance ruler" is a method of assessment where a patient is asked to indicate on a ruler or scale, where 0 is no importance and 10 is extreme importance, how important it is to him or her to make a change. While it may be tempting to ask patients why they are not at a 10 on the scale, this question elicits the opposite of change talk (i.e., reasons why they do *not* see it as extremely important). Instead, to elicit change talk, the clinician asks the patient to explain what made him or her pick a particular number (other than zero), as this represents the motivation the patient *does* have, by saying:

> "You picked a 3, so you do place at least a little bit of importance on this. What makes it at least a little bit important to you?"

Elaborating, querying extremes, and looking back and forward

Examples of each of these methods of fostering change talk are provided below. Querying extremes and looking back and forward are used to have the patient look beyond current obstacles to envisage how things *might be* in order to elicit change talk. Requesting elaboration is useful because it is quite common for patients to respond to a clinician's question about something like the advantages of making a change with one broad item, for example:

> "... it would improve my health ..."

An intuitive MI clinician will not simply move on but will rather ask for more detail and/or ask for additional advantages. When used in conjunction with reflective listening, a great deal more change talk tends to be expressed (Table 4.3).

Table 4.3. Examples of elaborating, querying extremes, and looking back and forward.

Elaborating	"In what ways? What else?" (Regarding reasons for change)
Querying extremes	"In the long run what concerns you the most?"
	"How much do you know about what can happen?"
	"What's the best outcome you could possibly imagine?"
Looking back and forward	"Do you remember a time when things were going well for you? What has changed?"
	"How do you want things to be 10 years from now?"

Exploring goals and values

One of the particularly useful methods of eliciting change talk is the exploration of goals and values. Goals and values are at the heart of an individual's own (or "internal") reasons for making behavior changes. Eliciting these and asking patients to consider their current behavior or proposed behavior change in light of the values can be a powerful. This method provides a means of developing discrepancy and eliciting change talk. For example, a clinician might ask:

> "What are the things that are most important to you?"

and then follow up with:

> "How do these goals/values relate to your smoking/eating/oral health behaviors/etc.?"

RESPONDING TO CHANGE TALK

Once change talk has been elicited, the goal in MI is to reinforce and encourage more change talk. Having said that, it is nevertheless important to recognize that because patients are typically ambivalent when they start talking about change, they are often prompted to talk about their concerns and why they cannot or do not want to change. An excessive focus on change by the clinician without acknowledging patient concerns is likely to prompt patients to start emphasizing barriers that clinicians commonly recognize as "resistance." Effectively reinforcing and encouraging change talk requires sensitivity to the patient's global perspective and state of ambivalence.

Table 4.4. Examples of responding to change talk.

Elaborate change talk	"What else are you concerned about?"
	"Are there any other advantages of changing that you see?"
Reflect and summarize change talk	"You feel that there could be some benefits to changing."
	"Changing would be really hard for you but you do worry about your health."
Affirm change talk	"I think you're right about that."
	"It's important to you to be a good parent."

Table 4.4 provides examples of methods of responding to change talk that reinforce and encourage further discussion. The second example illustrates how reflections and summaries can be used to acknowledge ambivalence, while also facilitating change talk. The key in this example is that the statement begins with an acknowledgement of ambivalence but ends with a reflection of change talk. By ending on change talk, the effect is to encourage elaboration of that aspect of the reflection. Advanced MI clinicians commonly use these types of reflections (as well as eliciting questions) to bring the conversation back on course when needed and to maintain momentum. While there is certainly purpose in the way the clinician chooses to make reflections, we rely on the patient's own statements and aspirations to move the conversation forward. "Cheerleading" (insincere and exaggerated responses of support), maneuvering, or manipulating are not part of MI because the impetus for change emerges from the patient's own sense of discrepancy.

Responding to resistance

By now, it should be clear that in MI "resistance" is seen as a reflection of patient ambivalence. In other words, resistance is typical and a normal expression of ambivalence. The key to responding to resistance is to "roll with it" rather than "pushing against it" and thus getting into an argument or debate. A number of methods are available for accomplishing this goal and these are outlined with the examples in Table 4.5.

The value of the skill of reflecting is highlighted again in Table 4.5, as the first three methods involve the use of reflections. The *simple reflection* is a powerful and uncomplicated way of rolling with resistance because, by definition, it avoids an argument (i.e., it is impossible to argue when you are restating what the other person has said). Clinicians sometimes express concern

Table 4.5. Examples of methods of rolling with resistance.

Simple reflection	Patient: "I really don't think I'm ready to make a change." Clinician: "You think that now is not a good time to make a change."
Amplified reflection	Patient: "Well, I really enjoy smoking, and frankly it just doesn't seem to be causing me much of a problem right now." Clinician: "You're not seeing any problems at all with your smoking."
Double-sided reflection	Clinician: "On the one hand you feel that it will be really hard to change because of how much you enjoy candy, but on the other hand you recognize there would be a lot of benefits, not just for your teeth and gums but also for your weight."
Agreement with a twist	Clinician: "Well, you're right, flossing can be time consuming and a hassle, but for most people so is dental treatment. It's sort of a trade-off between flossing and dental treatment."
Emphasizing personal choice and control	Clinician: "I notice you're a smoker and I'd like to talk to you about that if you would be willing. I promise I do not want to nag you or make you feel bad about being a smoker. The choice to smoke is completely up to you, but I would like to gain a better understanding of how you feel about your smoking."
Reframing	Clinician: "You feel like ice cream and candy is a way to treat yourself, but in the long run you are also treating yourself to a lot of pain and expense."
Coming alongside/ siding with the negative	Clinician: "You see absolutely no way to make a change and no possible way that I could help."
Shift focus	Clinician: "Well it sounds like you are quite doubtful about the information you have been provided and whether it really applies to you. Let's switch gears and talk about the concerns that you do have."

that by reflecting they are agreeing or acquiescing to something that may not be in the best interest of the patient. However, it is crucial to keep in mind that reflecting does not constitute agreement or approval. A reflection is meant to be a statement about what the patient said *without* any judgment (i.e., neither approval nor disapproval). Reflecting simply communicates an understanding of the patient's perspective. Ironically, by simply reflecting and avoiding an argument the clinician is therefore actually more likely to be able to influence the patient than when he or she disagrees and tries to persuade or convince the patient.

Amplified reflections are different from simple reflections in that they overstate or amplify the patient's resistance. Typically, this exaggeration of the patient's ambivalence will have the effect of the patient switching, at least briefly, to the side of change, for example, by saying:

"Well it's not that I don't see *any* benefit to change, it's just that ..."

In our experience this phenomenon is part of the broader matter of ambivalence and empathy. To the extent that patients feel that the clinician does not understand that it is hard to change, and/or that they have good reasons for doing what they are doing, patients will keep emphasizing these points. To the extent that patients feel that the clinician empathizes with their reasons for not changing, they will be willing to talk about their desire to change.

One useful way of capturing both sides of the ambivalence is with the third type of reflection: *the double-sided reflection.* This allows the clinician to reflect change talk while also acknowledging ambivalence. As noted earlier, a reflection that ends with the change talk component will invariably prompt further discussion in that direction.

Beyond reflections, there are various other means of responding to resistance. *Agreement with a twist* involves agreeing but with some variation or redirection in order to continue the focus on change. *Emphasizing personal choice and control* involves reminding the patient that ultimately the decision to change rests with him or her. The clinician can serve as a catalyst for discussion and consideration, but ultimately the patient is in charge of his or her own life. Affirming patients' autonomy can go a long way to reducing their fear that they will be pressed into doing something they don't want to do. When patients perceive less pressure for a particular outcome, they tend to be less resistant and more likely to be open to all the options.

Reframing involves changing the patient's perspective on something that he or she expresses. For example, a patient's repeated failures can be reframed as a sign of high motivation or persistence. *Coming alongside or siding with the negative* is a more extreme version of an amplified reflection in that the clinician completely agrees with the patient's resistant position (e.g., that change is pointless or hopeless). In a similar fashion to an amplified reflection, this can sometimes prompt the patient to budge from an extreme position of resistance to change to one of greater ambivalence. However, as it is possible that the patient will simply agree, this is a higher risk strategy that is best undertaken as a last resort.

Perhaps a more pragmatic approach is to simply *shift focus*. When it is clear that there is simply too much resistance to proceed in the same direction, the wisest course of action may be to simply shift focus and seek some common ground elsewhere. Clinicians can sometimes get caught up feeling that they must convince a patient of the merits of a particular argument for change, but often the argument is beside the point because what really matters is the reasons the *patient* sees for changing. Exploring that possibility, or at least preserving rapport for another discussion on another day, may be far more successful for a long-term relationship.

Enhancing confidence

While the heart of MI is focused on fostering motivation for change, it is clear that behavior change requires both the motivation to change as well as the confidence to make that change (Bandura 1997). Low confidence can undermine high motivation or importance. In MI, similar methods are used to foster motivation and confidence. Below, we describe a variety of methods used to enhance confidence, and in Table 4.6, we provide examples.

One way to enhance confidence is by using *evocative questions*. These questions help the patient to think about or visualize how the change might take place or reflect on what gives him or her confidence. The *confidence ruler* can be a useful tool for this purpose. This is the same as the "importance ruler" described at the beginning of this chapter except that the focus changes from importance to confidence. The goal of using the confidence ruler is to elicit "confidence talk."

The following provides an exercise using the confidence ruler to illustrate how this might work:

If you will, take a moment and think about a behavior change that you would like to make in your own life. It could be anything from quitting smoking, to eating better, exercising regularly, or getting more sleep; really anything. Now, focusing on that behavior, please answer the following question:

On a scale of 1 to 10, with 10 being very confident, how confident are you that you can change?

---

0 1 2 3 4 5 6 7 8 9 10

Not at all   Somewhat   Very

Chances are that you selected a number greater than zero. Let's say you selected a 1, 2, 3, or an even greater number, indicating that you have at least some confidence—what gives you that degree of confidence? Take a moment and reflect on the confidence that you have for making this change. Now that you've thought a bit about the confidence you already have, please consider the following question. What would need to happen for you to get from whatever number you picked to a somewhat higher number? Take a moment and reflect on what would really need to be different for you to feel more confident.

Table 4.6. Examples of methods to enhance confidence.

Evocative questions	"How might you go about making this change?" "What gives you some confidence that you can do this?"
Reviewing past success	"I quit smoking before when I was pregnant, so I think I could quit again if I set my mind to it."
Personal strengths and supports	"What difficult changes have you made in the past? What enabled you to do that? How might those strengths help with this?" "Who has helped you before? How could they help this time?"
Giving information and advice	Elicit: "If it's OK with you, I'd like to share some information that I think you might find useful. What have you been told about the benefits of avoiding sugary foods?" Provide: "You're right about that, but also … So one possibility that many patients tell me is helpful is to … ; another is to …" Elicit: "What do you think about that? Do any of those options sound like something that would work for you?"
Reframing	"You're disappointed because you quit for so long but then lapsed when your father died. But the good news is that this means you really know how to quit. Lots of my patients wish they could quit but haven't figured out how to get past the initial cravings. It sounds like the challenge is to build on that to learn how to avoid a relapse when something catastrophic occurs."
Hypothetical change	"What if you were a completely healthy eater. How would that have happened?"
Reinforce confidence talk	"It sounds like you do have some confidence that you could do this."

MOTIVATIONAL INTERVIEWING (MI) AND ITS BASIC TOOLS

The point of the exercise is to demonstrate how the ruler and follow-up questions can be used to elicit and enhance "confidence talk." After the first question, there are two key questions that accomplish this. The first is:

> "What gives you that degree of confidence?"

We find that this question is very counterintuitive, as most clinicians want to know:

> "Why are you not at a 10?"

and then move into problem-solving mode. In MI, there is recognition that individuals mostly have at least some degree of confidence that can be highlighted and enhanced. The second key question then moves the conversation into the issue of barriers to confidence but is phrased in terms of solutions, by asking:

> "What would it take to get you higher?"

rather than problems:

> "Why are you not a 10?"

Of course, the MI clinician would also be likely to follow up on each of these questions with reflective listening in order to encourage even more confidence talk.

Often patients have made attempts to change or had some form of success in the past. *Reviewing past success* can be valuable for identifying what strategies might be helpful for building confidence. Patients often fail to recognize that even if they succeeded with a change temporarily, something helped them to achieve even that temporary change.

Another method of fostering confidence is to *elicit or emphasize personal strengths* of the patient. A personal strength can be nearly any trait, but by affirming or highlighting it, the patient may see that it could contribute to success in his or her efforts to change. Similarly, successes in one area of life suggest strengths that could be applied to changes in other areas of the patient's life.

MOTIVATIONAL INTERVIEWING (MI) AND ITS BASIC TOOLS

Often patients become bogged down with obstacles, making it useful to consider *hypothetical change* that goes beyond them. Patients are prompted to envisage the change having "magically" taken place and then to think how that might have actually occurred. *Brainstorming*, where a number of potential solutions are generated without allowing any negative evaluation, can also be effective in fostering confidence through more creative solutions.

Clinicians can also often foster confidence by *providing information and advice*. Because in MI the goal is avoid the expert role, there are specific steps that can be taken to avoid the "expert trap." The goal should be to avoid providing advice unless desired by the patient. When the patient asks for advice, the desire is clear, but if the clinician suspects the patient may be interested, the clinician might ask permission to provide information or advice. When information is provided, it is recommended that it is offered "neutrally" in a form such as:

> "Research indicates …"

or:

> "Many of my patients tell me …"

or:

> "This may not fit for you, but …"

rather than:

> "I recommend …"

or:

> "I have found …"

This strategy avoids linking the information to the clinician, freeing the patient to reject the information without "rejecting the clinician."

Regardless of the method used to foster confidence, the overall goal should be to *reinforce "confidence talk."* As with change talk, the goal in MI is to have the patient do the thinking and talking, and the more he or she can be encouraged to talk about confidence to change, the better (Table 4.6).

Strengthening commitment

Once patients are motivated and have some confidence, they may be ready to make a commitment to change (or at least to try to change). The challenge in this phase is to accurately gauge the level of the patient's readiness in order to avoid seeking commitment too soon (which will usually result in increased resistance) or dwelling too long on motivation and missing a chance to move forward with a plan to change. In fact, there is some evidence that MI can be counterproductive for patients ready to make a change, so there is reason to be concerned about excessive exploration of motivation and confidence (Ashton 2006).

Signs of readiness to change include decreased resistance, greater calmness or resolve, increased change talk, questions about change, signs of envisaging the potential problems and benefits of change, and any small steps toward change. At this point, a summary that describes the clinician's impression of the key elements of the discussion can be useful to facilitate the transition. A clinician can summarize both the pros and cons, perhaps emphasizing the reasons for change, and then follow up with a key open question designed to facilitate the "next step." Some examples of key questions are:

"What changes, if any, would you consider making?"

"Reflecting on our discussion, what would be the next step?"

"It sounds like you don't want things to stay the same. What would you like to do?"

Negotiating a plan for change

Once the patient is sufficiently committed to change, the clinician can begin the final phase of MI: to develop a plan for change. Simple behavioral changes (e.g., brushing morning and night) may not require the development of a detailed plan, but complex behavior changes (e.g., smoking cessation) are best tackled with a formal plan.

A great way to help patients to strengthen their commitment to making the behavior change is to help them to see all the reasons, supports, and possible barriers to change in one place. One idea for doing so is to have patients

My reasons for making this change are:

To save my teeth

To feel better about my appearance

My plan is to (list specific steps/actions):

Talk to my doctor about quitting smoking

Brush twice a day and floss every night

Some possible barriers and how I could handle them:

Obstacle to change   Ways to address obstacle

Bad moods when I stop smoking   _Ask Doc about nicotine replacement_

Forgetting to floss   _Put reminder note on mirror_

Figure 4.2. Change plan worksheet.

complete a worksheet something like the one in Figure 4.2 (adapted from Miller and Rollnick 2002).

A word of caution about this phase: the temptation can sometimes be to forget the core MI principles and jump into the expert role by drawing up the clinician's ideal plan. However, in order for the plan to be effective for the patient, the MI approach continues to emphasize allowing the patient to take the lead. The clinician should try to facilitate the development of a plan that the patient believes will work for him or her.

The first step in this phase is to help the patient identify the specific goals that the plan should achieve. Goals should be clearly specified in terms that can easily be used to determine whether or not each goal has been achieved. Goals also need to be achievable or realistic in the patient's current circumstances. Sometimes there may be need to decide among a number of goals regarding what the priority should be. The clinician should facilitate the patient's consideration of these matters and provide input when appropriate in an MI style.

The next step is to consider how the patient can achieve the goal by developing a plan. Again, the key here is to first encourage the patient to generate ideas and potential solutions. The clinician can add or shape these ideas and in certain circumstances might offer some options for the patient to choose from. Again, elicit specific details, by asking:

> "What exactly will you do?"

> "How can you get this started?"

> "When will this occur?"

or:

> "Who could help?"

These questions will help the patient to develop a clear, well-thought-out plan that he or she can actually implement. The clinician can summarize the plan at the end to ensure that it is clearly understood, for example, by saying:

> "So if I have this right the plan is to ..."

Once agreed, the final step is to elicit commitment:

> "Does this sound like something you want to do?"

The clinician should pay close attention to the patient's response for signs of ambivalence, for example, by hearing the patient say:

> "Yeah, I guess so."

If the patient expresses hesitation, then the ambivalence should be explored using the motivational methods described earlier, by saying:

> "Sounds like you're not quite sure you want to do this."

Ideally, the patient will agree to commit to the plan and, if appropriate, follow-up should be arranged to see how it goes and to provide any further assistance necessary.

SUMMARY

In closing, we'd like to re-emphasize the point made earlier that MI is at heart a style, a way of interacting with patients, that if done properly often leads to enhanced motivation for targeted behavior change. It takes a lot of practice and is often harder than it looks! Nevertheless, research indicates non-counsellors can be effective when using MI, and each new patient represents an opportunity to work on the skills. We also encourage clinicians to focus less on whether their patients actually change (many individual and environmental factors influence a patient's ultimate behavior) and instead on using MI to have meaningful conversations with their patients. In time, the positive relationship that is developed and the seeds for change that are planted may well blossom into full-fledged health behavior change.

REFERENCES

Almomani, F., T. Brown, et al. (2009). Effects of an oral health promotion program in people with mental Illness. *J Dent Res* 88(7):648–652.

Amrhein, P.C., W.R. Miller, et al. (2003). Client commitment language during motivational interviewing predicts drug use outcomes. *J Consult Clin Psychol* 71(5):862–878.

Ashton, M. (ed.). (2006). My way or yours? *Drug and Alcohol Findings* 15:22–29.

Bandura, A. (1997). *Self-Efficacy: The Exercise of Control.* New York: W.H. Freeman.

Borrelli, B., S. Novak, et al. (2005). Home health care nurses as a new channel for smoking cessation treatment: Outcomes from project CARES (Community-nurse Assisted Research and Education on Smoking). *Prev Med* 41(5–6):815–821.

Bowen, D., C. Ehret, et al. (2002). Results of an adjunct dietary intervention program in the Women's Health Initiative. *J Am Diet Assoc* 102(11):1631–1637.

Burke, B.L., H. Arkowitz, et al. (2003). The efficacy of motivational interviewing: A meta-analysis of controlled clinical trials. *J Consult Clin Psychol* 71(5):843–861.

Burke, B.L., C.W. Dunn, et al. (2004). The emerging evidence base for motivational interviewing: A meta-analytic and qualitative inquiry. *J Cognitive Psychotherapy* 18(4):309–322.

Butler, C.C., S. Rollnick, et al. (1999). Motivational consulting versus brief advice for smokers in general practice: A randomized trial. *Br J General Practice* 49:611–616.

Centers for Disease Control and Prevention. (2002). Cigarette smoking among adults—United States. *Morbidity & Mortality Weekly Report* 51:642–645.

Curry, S.J. (2003). Youth tobacco cessation: Filling the gap between what we do and what we know. *Am J Health Behav* 27 Suppl 2:S99–102.

Hettema, J., J. Steele, et al. (2005). Motivational interviewing. *Annual Review of Clinical Psychology* 1:91–111.

Jönsson, B., K. Ohrn, et al. (2009). An individually tailored treatment programme for improved oral hygiene: Introduction of a new course of action in health education for patients with periodontitis. *Int J Dent Hyg* 7(3):166–175.

Mhurchu, C.N., B.M. Margetts, et al. (1998). Randomized clinical trial comparing the effectiveness of two dietary interventions for patients with hyperlipidaemia. *Clin Sci (Lond)* 95(4):479–487.

Miller, W.R. (1983). Motivational interviewing with problem drinkers. *Behavioral Psychotherapy* 11:147–172.

Miller, W.R., and S. Rollnick (eds.). (1991). *Motivational Interviewing: Preparing People for Change.* New York: Guilford Press.

Miller, W.R., and S. Rollnick (eds.). (2002). *Motivational Interviewing: Preparing People for Change,* 2nd ed. New York: Guilford Press.

Pbert, L., S.K. Osganian, et al. (2006). A school nurse-delivered adolescent smoking cessation intervention: A randomized controlled trial. *Prev Med* 43(4):312–320.

Resnicow, K., C. DiIorio, et al. (2002). Motivational interviewing in health promotion: It sounds like something is changing. *Health Psychol* 21(5):444–451.

Resnicow, K., A. Jackson, et al. (2001). A motivational interviewing intervention to increase fruit and vegetable intake through black churches: Results of the Eat for Life trial. *Am J Public Health* 91(10):1686–1693.

Richards, A., K.K. Kattelmann, et al. (2006). Motivating 18- to 24-year-olds to increase their fruit and vegetable consumption. *J Am Diet Assoc* 106(9):1405–1411.

Rollnick, S., and W.R. Miller. (1995). What is motivational interviewing? *Behavioral and Cognitive Psychotherapy* 23:325–334.

Rubak, S., A. Sandbaek, et al. (2005). Motivational interviewing: A systematic review and meta-analysis. *Br J Gen Pract* 55(513):305–312.

Ryan, R.M., and E.L. Deci. (2000). Self-determination theory and the facilitation of intrinsic motivation, social development, and well-being. *Am Psychol* 55(1):68–78.

Soria, R., A. Legido, et al. (2006). A randomised controlled trial of motivational interviewing for smoking cessation. *Br J Gen Pract* 56(531):768–774.

Valanis, B., E. Lichtenstein, et al. (2001). Maternal smoking cessation and relapse prevention during health care visits. *Am J Prev Med* 20(1):1–8.

Wakefield, M., I. Olver, et al. (2004). Motivational interviewing as a smoking cessation intervention for patients with cancer: Randomized controlled trial. *Nurs Res* 53(6):396–405.

Weinstein, P., R. Harrison, et al. (2006). Motivating mothers to prevent caries: Confirming the beneficial effect of counseling. *J Am Dent Assoc* 137(6):789–793.

Weinstein, P., R. Harrison, et al. (2004). Motivating parents to prevent caries in their young children: One-year findings. *J Am Dent Assoc* 135(6):731–738.

Williams, G.C., R.M. Frankel, et al. (2000). Research on relationship-centered care and healthcare outcomes from the Rochester biopsychosocial program: A self-determination theory integration. *Families, Systems & Health* 18:79–90.

MOTIVATIONAL INTERVIEWING (MI) AND ITS BASIC TOOLS

CHAPTER 5
BRIEF INTERVENTIONS IN PROMOTING HEALTH BEHAVIOR CHANGE

Anne Koerber

Key Points of This Chapter

- Brief interventions could be effective in helping patients along their continuum to change while taking up 5–15 minutes of a dental appointment.
- Brief interventions should target three main issues of health behavior change: (1) assessing motives, (2) raising awareness, and (3) supporting change.
- Behavior change itself may not be the best goal for one single brief intervention. Each brief intervention may accomplish one simple step toward behavior change by a cumulative effect over time.
- In brief interventions, the health history form, open-ended questions, and the readiness scales are used to assess the patients' views of behavior change.
- In brief interventions, asking permission, expressing concern or empathy, or linking to clinical findings before raising awareness of health issues helps to build or maintain rapport with the patient.
- To maintain rapport in brief interventions, clinicians ask for permission, express empathy, or link to clinical findings while raising awareness of health issues with patients.
- Supporting patient change in brief interventions is achieved by (1) encouraging patient problem solving, (2) offering a set of strategies or options, and (3) planning steps for the change.

INTRODUCTION

As clinicians experience more pressure to use time effectively and maximize productivity, they seek briefer and more efficient techniques to influence behavior change in patients. While complex behavior changes cannot be expected to happen quickly, there are techniques that have been shown to facilitate change even when only a short amount of time is available. The focus of this chapter is on forming brief, effective interventions that may help patients along their continuum to change.

> Brief interventions could be effective in helping patients along their continuum to change while taking up 5–15 minutes of a dental appointment.

The following content relies mainly on Motivational Interviewing principles described by Miller and Rollnick and others, which have been adapted to dental situations (Miller and Rollnick 2002; Rollnick et al. 1999; Rollnick 2002). For the purpose of this chapter, brief interventions are defined as those that could be effective while taking up 5–15 minutes of a dental appointment with a patient.

> Brief interventions should target three main issues of health behavior change: (1) assessing motives, (2) raising awareness, and (3) supporting change.

The over-arching structure of how the clinician can facilitate health behavior change with a patient is the same for brief interventions as for longer interventions: first, if the patient doesn't recognize the importance of a change, the clinician focuses on helping the patient see the importance; second, if the patient recognizes the importance of a change but doesn't feel able to make the change, the clinician focuses on helping the patient discover how to make the change. In summary, brief interventions address three possible issues: (1) assessing motives, (2) raising awareness, and (3) supporting change. As mentioned and discussed in the previous chapters of this book, the clinician must take care to avoid argumentation and maintain rapport while addressing these issues (Rollnick 2002).

USING A PATIENT-CENTERED APPROACH

A patient-centered approach requires addressing change from the patient's point of view. The clinician has a set of goals to offer the patient, but in order to be effective the clinician partners with the patient, rather than taking an authoritative, directive stance. With the limited amount of time available to repair breaches of empathy, avoiding or rolling with resistance may be even more essential in brief interventions than longer interventions. Although it isn't intuitively obvious, using a patient-centered Motivational Interviewing approach saves time over more traditional educational or persuasive approaches because it is less likely to create resistance.

As discussed in chapter 4, Motivational Interviewing techniques are focused on understanding patient motives and ambivalences rather than imparting information or persuading a patient. As soon as the focus is set on the patient's motives, or on what the patient wants in life, rather than on what the clinician thinks the patient ought to do, the sooner the patient will engage in change (Miller and Rollnick 2002).

Righting reflex

Brief interventions require self-control from the clinician. When time is limited, the concerned clinician may be tempted to pressure the patient to commit to a change. As introduced in chapters 3 and 4, Miller and Rollnick refer to this as the "righting reflex" (Miller and Rollnick 2002). In brief interventions, the clinicians tend to "put things right" by pushing the patient in the desired direction. Unfortunately, this risks eliciting resistance from the patient. It is only human nature to push back when being pushed. If a clinician tries to force the patient to commit to change before being ready, the patient is likely to feel resentful and misunderstood. Furthermore, if clinicians respond to time pressures by talking more than listening, their ability to understand the patient's point of view is reduced. To be effective, brief interventions require clinicians to control their instinct or desire to push. Even during a brief intervention, clinicians accept that the patient is in control of any change that is made.

Fortunately, dental visits often occur frequently over time, allowing dental clinicians to build on past appointments and allowing behavior change to emerge on its own timeline. Research suggests that frequency of contact increases the likelihood that health counseling interventions will be effective (Rigotti et al. 2007).

Goals of brief interventions

Brief interventions are usually able to be short because the goals of one appointment are limited, but not because patient talk is limited. Behavior

Behavior change itself may not be the best goal for one single brief intervention. Each brief intervention may accomplish one simple step toward behavior change by a cumulative effect over time.

change itself may not be the best goal for one single brief intervention. Only relatively simple steps toward behavioral changes will be accomplished in one brief intervention. Additionally, clinicians who understand how to limit the goals of each brief appointment feel less need to push the patient, are more aware of what they can accomplish in a brief amount of time, and therefore feel less frustration with patients.

ASSESSING MOTIVES

Assessment of the patient's readiness to change involves learning about the importance of change for the patient and how confident the patient feels to make the change (Miller and Rollnick 2002). When time is limited, the first of these two is most important to uncover: why might a patient feel it is important to make a change?

In brief interventions, the use of a health history form, open-ended questions, and the readiness scales is suggested for assessing the patients' views of behavior change.

The clinician can't expect that a patient is motivated by some abstract wish for good health (Rollnick et al. 1999). As noted in previous chapters, something important to one patient may not be important to another. Likewise, that which is important to the clinician may not be important to the patient. When assessing importance, the clinician seeks to discover the patient's specific motivators and values, in order to link them to the desired behavior change. We describe here three ways to assess motives expeditiously. The first is through the health history form. The second is through open-ended questions, and the third is by using the readiness scale.

Health history form

The health history form is an excellent method to obtain information on patient motivation by asking about the chief complaint and motives for oral health. The question could be phrased as:

> "What would you like to get from dental treatment during your time with us?"

or:

> "What goals do you have for your teeth and mouth in the long run?"

The clinician can then apply that information to the desired behavior. For example, if it was noted on the health history form that the patient wants pretty teeth and sweet breath, the clinician can use that information to target better attention to oral hygiene or to target smoking cessation. Sometimes, the information obtained from the health history form is sufficient to understand a patient's motivation, and the clinician may immediately move to the next step of supporting change.

Open-ended questions

The second method of obtaining information about motives and thus importance is by using open-ended questions about the patient's goals, feelings, and desires. Rollnick and co-authors suggest that skillful asking involves short, simply worded questions that feel part of normal conversation to the patient (Rollnick et al. 2007).

Here are a few examples:

> "Please tell me how you feel about quitting smoking."

> "In your opinion, what are the pros and cons to you of quitting smoking?"

> "I wonder what your hopes and goals are for your daughter's mouth and teeth as she grows up."

> "Regarding flossing and brushing, would you tell me what reasons you have for keeping your teeth clean?"

> "What would you like to get from a new set of dentures?"

> "Would you mind sharing with me what you have heard about gum disease?"

The use of open-ended questions was thoroughly described in chapter 3. It may come as a surprise to the reader that asking open-ended questions is suggested as a technique for brief interventions. Contrary to common thinking, open-ended questions are most efficient for obtaining complex narrative information about patient views and opinions, knowledge of which are essential for helping a client change (Rollnick et al. 2007). The clinicians can use their listening skills to uncover and then clarify the patient's goals.

Clinicians may avoid using open-ended questions out of fear of patients talking on and on, sometimes about unrelated elements. However, the vast majority of patients will respond to an open-ended question by providing considerable information about their motivation. In addition, allowing patients to tell the story in their own words develops rapport. For patients who are too talkative, chatty, or rambling, clinicians can gently ask permission to interrupt when they have heard enough to clarify the motives. By summarizing what they have heard and redirecting the patient, they will be able to keep the intervention focused and brief.

Readiness scales

The third method of obtaining information about motivation to change is to use the readiness scales consisting of (1) the importance scale, and (2) the confidence scale as described by Rollnick, Mason, and Butler (Rollnick et al. 1999).

First, the importance scale consists of three questions. For example:

---

1. "On a scale of 1 to 10, where 10 is absolutely important and 1 is not at all important, how would you rate the importance of (quitting smoking, flossing your teeth regularly, preventing more tooth decay in your child, etc.)?"
2. "Why did you rate it as (X) instead of 1?"
3. "Why did you rate it as (X) instead of 10?"

Note that question 2 reveals the patient's motives, and question 3 reveals the patient's ambivalence.

Second, the confidence scale consists of the following questions:

> 1. "If you were convinced that (quitting smoking, flossing your teeth regularly, preventing more tooth decay in your child, etc.) were very important, on a scale of 1 to 10, how confident are you that you could do it? One means not at all confident and 10 means completely confident."
> 2. "Why did you rate it as (X) instead of 1?"
> 3. "Why did you rate it as (X) instead of 10?"

Note here that question 2 reveals a patient's strengths to make the change, and question 3 reveals the barriers. Using this series of questions, the clinician can form a rather complete picture of a patient's position regarding change within a short amount of time.

Three methods of assessing motives have been discussed so far: questions on the health history, open-ended questions, and use of the readiness scales. The use of the readiness scales may be all that can be accomplished in one brief intervention. At this point, therefore, the clinician may end the intervention by summarizing the patient's goals and motives, mentioning any possible next steps, and taking notes to facilitate another brief intervention at a subsequent appointment.

RAISING AWARENESS

Once motives are known, the clinician can use that information to motivate a patient to make a change. However, in some cases, the clinician will need to raise the patient's awareness of the problem. Periodontal disease, oral mucosal lesions, tobacco use, diabetes, and infant nursing practices are examples of issues that patients may not spontaneously identify as important in a dental office. In addition, patients may be aware of issues such as tobacco use that they know are considered "bad" by health professionals, but about which they have little personal concern.

For brief appointments, one way of handling patient lack of motivation is to express concern, empathize with the patient's position, and ask for permission to check in with the patient periodically and see if he or she has become more interested in change. This method essentially acknowledges the current lack of motivation and makes no attempt to change that situation beyond an expression of concern. Alternatively, the clinician may choose to raise the patient's awareness of the importance of the issue.

When raising awareness, it is important to introduce the subject with respect for the patient's autonomy. This can be done in a number of ways, but probably the most direct is to ask for permission to discuss the issue. For example, the clinician might say:

> "Could we talk a bit about the condition of your gums?"

When introducing a new subject, it is also helpful to link it with a clinical finding or with a motive that the patient has already identified as important, which demonstrates to the patient why the subject is being raised. If this step is not done, the patient may see the intervention as generic and not pertaining specifically to him or her. Consider the difference in impact on a patient between saying:

> "I always recommend that people avoid eating sugar between meals."

or saying:

> "You have new cavities each time I see you. I wonder if you would be willing to consider ways of avoiding getting cavities."

When raising awareness, it is often most efficient to focus on objective risks of the exposure instead of the patient's unfavorable behavior (Rollnick 2002). This approach avoids blaming while still emphasizing the importance of the issue. In addition to focusing on risk, mentioning the beneficial aspects of change without being too prescriptive conveys a sense of hope and increases the patient's self-efficacy. Table 5.1 contrasts methods of raising a patient's awareness about various issues, showing the benefits of the points just addressed.

Giving information versus raising awareness

In brief interventions, it is important to provide information in the most effective manner possible in the short amount of time available. It may help with efficiency if the clinician thinks of the process as raising awareness instead of providing information or "educating" the patient. Because people tend to remember and assimilate information better when it is interesting to them, information provided in brief interventions should be designed to engage the patient's interest. By definition, this includes any information already requested by the patient. In the absence of other cues from the patient,

Table 5.1. Comparison of potential and improved interventions to raise awareness.

Potential Intervention	Analysis of the Intervention	Improved Intervention
You should quit chewing tobacco.	Focuses on "bad" behavior instead of risk, and doesn't link the issue to the patient's condition or goals.	I know your primary interest is in making your smile prettier. But may we talk about this rough, white area under your lip? It is a reaction of your mouth to the tobacco.
I recommend you quit chewing tobacco.	Better than the previous statement, and it has the advantage of being direct, but it doesn't ask permission.	May we talk about chewing tobacco?
Chewing tobacco causes cancer.	Focuses on cause instead of risk or beneficial aspects of change.	You will lower your risk of getting mouth cancer if you quit chewing tobacco.
I'm sorry to say I'm seeing gum disease here. Gum disease is caused by plaque on the teeth. Plaque is the same sticky bacterial film that causes tooth decay. The bacteria actually cause an infection in your gums, because you aren't cleaning your teeth properly.	Start with information on risk and the benefits of change. Too much peripheral information is given in this example. Focuses on "bad" behavior.	I'm concerned because I'm seeing gum disease here. There is an infection in your gums; if it continues, you risk losing some teeth. May we talk about some ways you could control that infection?
You need to stop letting your baby go to bed with the bottle now that her teeth have erupted. The milk pools on her teeth and causes cavities.	The focus is on "bad" behavior. Risk information is provided; the benefits of change should also be mentioned.	Would you be willing to go over some things you could do to reduce your baby's risk of getting cavities?

In brief interventions, asking permission, expressing concern or empathy, or linking to clinical findings before raising awareness of health issues all help to build or maintain rapport with the patient.

information about risk appears to be the most salient. When phrased correctly to demonstrate importance to the patient, it will also be the information most likely to be retained. Next to risk information, the most important information to provide is a sense of optimism, a sense that the patient can improve the situation. All other information, for example, about causes, disease processes, and treatments, is most appropriately provided only after the patient has shown an interest. In summary, information will not be effective if the patient doesn't assimilate it; and patients are unlikely to assimilate information if they don't understand why it is important to them. In brief interventions, less information is often more (Rollnick et al. 2007).

Conveying understanding

One of the most useful brief interventions a clinician can make is to convey understanding of the patient's situation. Building rapport is a key principle of Motivational Interviewing (Miller and Rollnick 2002) and a pillar of behavior change. Reflecting the patient's feelings or thoughts about an issue, often by noting both sides of a patient's ambivalence, shows understanding. When an intervention is made that conveys understanding, a climate of acceptance is created for the patient. Within this climate, the patient can relax, and he or she drops the need to engage in arguments or defensiveness, which is the first step toward problem solving with the patient.

To maintain rapport in brief interventions, clinicians ask for permission, express empathy, or link to clinical findings while raising awareness of health issues with patients.

Summarizing statements convey understanding and have the added effect of helping the patient clarify concerns to him- or herself and to the clinician, which in turn may help them both see what the next steps are. In brief interviews, the specific advantages to both reflecting and summarizing interventions are (1) they deepen the relationship with the patient, (2) they name and address problems, while (3) keeping the responsibility for the next step with the patient. It is probably good practice to end all brief interventions with a summarizing statement about the patient's position (Rollnick 2002). Table 5.2 reviews some examples of interventions to convey understanding.

Table 5.2. Examples of conveying understanding.

Reflections:

"I can understand that it's too stressful for you to quit smoking right now."

"You have found that the baby cries when you take the bottle away from her at night."

"You'd really like to find a way to quit, but you're worried that you can't do it."

Summarizing ambivalence:

"It feels too stressful for you to quit smoking right now, although you are concerned about your heart."

"It causes too many problems for you when the baby cries at night, so you don't feel you can keep withholding the bottle even though you are concerned about her teeth."

Summarizing to close a brief session:

"I hear that you aren't ready to consider quitting right now. May I check in with you about that next time I see you?"

"You are telling me that you've decided to cut down on your children's sugary foods. Will you call me next week and let me know how that is going?"

"OK, you are going to consider ways of helping yourself remember to floss between now and when I see you again next week. We can check out how that's going then.

SUPPORTING CHANGE

Supporting change is offered once a patient believes that a behavior change is needed. Patients may come to an appointment already knowing they need to change, or they may arrive at that belief after a series of appointments with the clinician. If the clinician assessment reveals that the patient agrees with the importance of change, the intervention needed is one to support change. The type of intervention needed depends on what kind of support the patient needs. When a patient has indicated that change is important, the next step is to explore what kind of help is needed to make that change.

One observed trap that clinicians run into with patients at this point, particularly when time is limited, is to be too directive or prescriptive. It helps the patients to adopt a new behavior if they see themselves as having a choice in the matter. As previous chapters in this book have emphasized, prescribing to a patient is liable to raise resistance. Furthermore, it encourages the patients to be dependent and passive regarding their own health, and to look to the clinician for solutions. Preferably, the clinician should be in the role of offering

> Supporting patient change in brief interventions is achieved by (1) encouraging patient problem solving, (2) offering a set of strategies or options, and (3) planning steps for the change.

options and helping a patient decide which options are best (Rollnick et al. 2007), rather than dictating the change. Broadly speaking, there are three categories of supporting patient change in a brief encounter: (1) encouraging patient problem solving, (2) offering a set of strategies, and (3) planning for the change.

Encouraging patient problem solving

Encouraging patient problem solving occurs when a clinician asks the patient to list his or her possible options, suggests that the patient remember what has helped in the past, or has the patient recall successes (Rollnick et al. 1999). This might be accompanied by providing the patient with literature or suggesting websites, or otherwise encouraging patient exploration and self-efficacy. A clinician may make suggestions to a patient in a manner to encourage self-efficacy by speaking in terms of what has worked for other patients, such as, "Some patients have found it helps to link flossing with something else they do regularly, like when they watch television at night" (Rollnick et al. 2007). This allows the clinician to make suggestions, while also acknowledging the patients' autonomy and their need to adapt the suggestion to their own situation.

Offering a set of strategies

When the clinician wants to encourage patient change sooner rather than later, offering a menu of strategies is a way of talking about change without being too prescriptive (Miller and Rollnick 2002; Rollnick et al. 1999). The intervention constitutes providing a patient with a list of behaviors or strategies that could help the situation. These interventions are also appropriate when the patients ask for their options. To help make interventions more efficient (and briefer), the clinician could develop and have on hand standard menus for frequently appearing situations. For example, a clinician could have available methods of reducing caries rates (specific for adults, infants, children, and adolescents), for reducing or controlling periodontal disease, for improving the appearance of a smile, for tobacco cessation, and so on.

Offering a set of options or strategies for change helps reduce resistance by allowing the patient to choose which behaviors he or she is ready to adopt at the moment. Furthermore, it encourages patient autonomy and responsibility by involving the patient directly in choices. Finally, it allows the patient to see the full range of options available without feeling pressured to engage in the most difficult first.

At the beginning of a brief intervention, the clinician could introduce the set of options, allow the patient to take time to review it and ask questions, and suggest the patient take the list home to think it over. An auxiliary could be made available for questions if the clinician needs to move on. If necessary, the options in the menu may be reviewed each time the patient comes in, and progress can be monitored and encouraged. For example, if a mother agrees on the importance of reducing her child's caries risk, she might choose a fluoride varnish at the first appointment and agree to daily oral hygiene with the child. She could return on the second appointment and discuss her progress or problems with providing daily oral hygiene. She and the clinician could then see if she was ready to consider reducing sugar intake or removing the bottle from the child outside of mealtimes.

One of the most helpful interventions a clinician can make for certain problems is to raise the patient's awareness of the option of more in-depth counselling. There are issues such as depression, anxiety, family problems, medication compliance, diabetic diet compliance, and alcohol or drug abuse that may affect oral health but probably require formal counselling in order to support change. In these cases, in addition to the other interventions discussed in this chapter, the clinician could choose to discuss referral for further counselling as an option with the patient. This could be suggested by making formal counselling one of the strategies listed on the menu, or by noting that other people have found formal counselling useful and asking for the patient's thoughts on that.

Planning for the change

Planning for change is a notably useful approach when the patient has made a decision to change and has an idea of what will be changed. In formal Motivational Interviewing, this is not a brief technique. Consequently, when the patient is planning to make structural changes in his or her life, such as dealing with addiction, shifting to a diabetic diet, or adjusting to chronic pain, planning for change likely requires formal counselling, which the clinician may prefer to refer to other professionals.

However, patients are often fully prepared in the dental office to make certain changes, such as flossing more frequently, using a softer toothbrush, or decreasing their sugar intake. In these cases, planning for the change is entirely possible during a brief intervention and will make it more likely that the change actually occurs (Gollwitzer and Sheeran 2006; Gollwitzer and Oettingen 2007). The intervention consists of asking the patient how and when he or she intends to engage in the behavior. This can be accompanied by a statement such as:

> "Many of our patients have found this works better if they think through the change here in the office, so they feel better prepared to do it at home."

Table 5.3 contains further examples.

Table 5.3. Examples of planning for change.

"Would you tell me where and when you will take these pills I've prescribed?"

"Studies show that people are more likely to floss if they plan when and where they will floss each day (Sniehotta et al. 2007). Could you tell me when and where you will floss for the next 2 weeks?"

"I've found people are more likely to be able to make a change if they think it through here. What are you going to do when you go home and your daughter wants the baby bottle between mealtimes?"

"Would you be willing to consider calling the surgeon right now to make an appointment to have that lesion examined?"

USE OF THE TELEPHONE FOR BRIEF INTERVENTIONS

Many studies of behavior change interventions have used the telephone as a convenient and brief method of encouraging or supporting patient change (Abdullah et al. 2005; An et al. 2006; Hanssen et al. 2007; Nitzke et al. 2007; Vanwormer et al. 2006; Wu et al. 2006). Telephone calls are used for checking in and for problem solving after patients have chosen to make a behavior change. Telephone calls have been used to follow up on smoking cessation, increasing exercise, and increasing fruit and vegetable intake, and to facilitate compliance with medications. They provide an opportunity for the patient to describe concerns and for the clinician to answer questions, indicate potential strategies, encourage patient problem solving, and otherwise support the patient in changing behavior. Dental offices often use telephone calls to follow up after surgical procedures, so follow-up for behavior change could be designed to fit into the office routine in a similar manner. This might be quite effective for checking in with patients to see how it is going with their flossing, for example.

The difficulty with telephone interventions is fitting them into the clinician's schedule. Busy clinicians may not be able to handle interruptions from patient phone calls. Telephone contact may be delegated to a member of the team, such as the dental assistant or receptionist. A practice team member such as an assistant or receptionist might be trained in proper behavior change techniques or may simply inquire about issues and then notify the dentist or hygienist if the patient wants to speak directly with the clinician. In multi-ethnic environments, team members of similar background as the patient may be helpful in facilitating patient change.

USE OF COMPUTERS FOR BRIEF INTERVENTIONS

Behavior change research has frequently examined the use of computers to assist patients in behavior change. This can be very efficient in facilitating behavior change because computers save clinician time. The computer intervention is designed to provide information to the patient in manageable "chunks," and a computer allows the patient to choose from menus the information he or she is interested in. The information usually includes risk information, other disease information, information on strategies to help change, and information on the benefits of possible behavior changes. Computers have the advantage of providing information without "pushing," entirely according to the patient's wishes, and can be effective (Block et al. 2000; Bussey-Smith and Rossen 2007; Neumann et al. 2006). After the computer intervention, the clinician may be able to limit the intervention to asking the patient what he or she decided to do and answering any further questions. The disadvantages, however, are many: the computer programs have to be purchased; they may not be available for oral health issues; space and computers must be provided for the intervention; and finally, they may not be useful if patients speak a non-standard language or are not literate. However, this kind of intervention shows promise for reaching larger numbers of patients if the proper programs can be developed for oral health situations.

GIVING BRIEF ADVICE

So far, we have discussed brief interventions that would be useful in an ongoing relationship with a patient. There are situations when it is unlikely that a patient will be seen again, but the clinician feels an obligation to provide information to the patient that might be helpful. Brief advice is used when only a few minutes are available to inform a patient about an issue. This is used in response to a patient question, because the clinician feels ethically bound to discuss it, or because the clinician feels it may be helpful to the patient. Rollnick suggests the goals that can be addressed with brief advice include demonstrating respect, communicating risk, providing information, and initiating thinking about change (in other words, raising awareness; Rollnick et al. 2007; Rollnick 2002).

Brief advice is characterized by bringing up risk information to the patient right away without assessing the patient's view of importance or confidence to change. An excellent method of initiating brief advice is to request permission to discuss the issue with the patient. Information about causes or details about the course of an illness are not to be discussed unless the patient asks. Instead, the information provided is focused toward risk and how a behavior change would reduce that risk. Rollnick suggests that the statement of advice should be followed by an open-ended invitation to the patient to respond to the advice, if time is available (Rollnick 2002). As a final step, the clinician listens closely and summarizes the patient's position, and may suggest a next step or ask the patient what the next step is.

WHEN BRIEF INTERVENTIONS ARE NOT APPROPRIATE

Brief interventions are unlikely to change behaviors that are highly entrenched in an existing lifestyle. In addition, there are some behaviors that dental professionals are not trained to treat, briefly or otherwise. Examples of such behaviors include heavy drinking, drug abuse, and bingeing, purging, or restricting food. In these cases, the brief intervention should be oriented toward helping the patient obtain counselling rather than helping the patient change behavior. Of course, the clinicians who lack training or interest may refer all sorts of behavioral issues to other professionals for further help.

BRINGING IT ALL TOGETHER

Brief interventions can assess, convey understanding, raise awareness, and support change. Any of these interventions are probably most effective if the clinician listens very closely to the patient and then summarizes the patient's position on the change. The clinician may also provide any information the patient asks for, or indicate options that might be helpful. The clinician may then ask the patient what the next step is, may suggest that the patient continue to consider options, or may ask the patient for permission to check in about the issue at his or her next appointment.

Brief multiple interventions are more effective when structured to build upon each other. The clinician could raise ongoing issues at each appointment by asking permission to follow up on the issue from the last appointment, while recognizing that there are other issues the patient may want to discuss instead. Open-ended questions are most likely to give the patient the opportunity to bring up any shift in attitude or behavior since the last appointment. If a particular change was discussed, the clinician could ask how that worked. If the patient was contemplating a change, the clinician could ask for his or her current thoughts about change. The subject might be reintroduced in some variation of the following:

"I'm curious how flossing has worked for you since I saw you last. Could we talk about that, or is there something else you wanted to discuss?"

"There were a few things we discussed last time about reducing Sally's risk for tooth decay. I remember we talked about the baby bottle, we talked about what kinds of drinks to give her, and we talked about fluoride. Could we continue to discuss tooth decay, or is there something else you would like to discuss today?"

"May I check with you about smoking?"

Multiple brief interventions will be most useful if the clinician makes notes about the patient's stage at the end of the last appointment and about any actions the patient agreed to take at that appointment. At the same time, the clinician should also keep in mind that the patient's situations and attitudes may change between appointments and not assume that his or her position is the same at any new appointment.

SUMMARY

In this chapter, we have shown how a clinician can provide brief behavioral change interventions for the purposes of assessment, raising awareness, supporting change, and conveying understanding. The keys to brief interventions are limiting the focus and goals of the appointment, keeping the interventions patient centered, avoiding argumentation or blame, and letting the patient take responsibility for whatever change is made. With these tools dental clinicians can, over time, help patients adopt more healthful behaviors.

REFERENCES

Abdullah, A.S., Y.W. Mak, et al. (2005). Smoking cessation intervention in parents of young children: A randomised controlled trial. *Addiction* 100(11):1731–1740.

An, L.C., S.H. Zhu, et al. (2006). Benefits of telephone care over primary care for smoking cessation: A randomized trial. *Arch Intern Med* 166(5):536–542.

Block, G., M. Miller, et al. (2000). An interactive CD-ROM for nutrition screening and counseling. *Am J Public Health* 90(5):781–785.

Bussey-Smith, K.L., and R.D. Rossen. (2007). A systematic review of randomized control trials evaluating the effectiveness of interactive computerized asthma patient education programs. *Ann Allergy Asthma Immunol* 98(6):507–516; quiz 516, 566.

Gollwitzer, P.M., and G. Oettingen. (2007). The role of goal setting and goal striving in medical adherence. In: L.L. Liu and D.C. Park, *Medical Adherence and Aging: Social and Cognitive Perspectives*. Washington, DC: American Psychological Association, 23–47.

Gollwitzer, P.M., and P. Sheeran. (2006). Implementation intentions and goal achievement: A meta-analysis of effects and processes. *Adv Exp Soc Psychol* 38:69–119.

Hanssen, T.A., J.E. Nordrehaug, et al. (2007). Improving outcomes after myocardial infarction: A randomized controlled trial evaluating effects of a telephone follow-up intervention. *Eur J Cardiovasc Prev Rehabil* 14(3):429–437.

Miller, W.R., and S. Rollnick (eds.). (2002). *Motivational Interviewing: Preparing People for Change*, 2nd ed. New York: Guilford Press.

Neumann, T., B. Neuner, et al. (2006). The effect of computerized tailored brief advice on at-risk drinking in subcritically injured trauma patients. *J Trauma* 61(4):805–814.

Nitzke, S., K. Kritsch, et al. (2007). A stage-tailored multi-modal intervention increases fruit and vegetable intakes of low-income young adults. *Am J Health Promot* 22(1):6–14.

Rigotti, N.A., M.R. Munafo, et al. (2007). Interventions for smoking cessation in hospitalised patients. *Cochrane Database Syst Rev* (3), CD001837.

Rollnick, S. (2002). Variations on a theme: Motivational interviewing and its adaptations. In: W.R. Miller and S. Rollnick, *Motivational Interviewing: Preparing People for Change*, 2nd ed. New York: Guilford Press, 270–283.

Rollnick, S., P. Mason, et al. (eds.). (1999). *Health Behavior Change: A Guide for Practitioners*. Edinburgh: Churchill Livingstone.

Rollnick, S., W.R. Miller, et al. (eds.). (2007). *Motivational Interviewing in Health Care*. New York: Guilford Press.

Sniehotta, F.F., V. Araujo Soares, et al. (2007). Randomized controlled trial of a one-minute intervention changing oral self-care behavior. *J Dent Res* 86(7):641–645.

Vanwormer, J.J., J.L. Boucher, et al. (2006). Telephone-based counseling improves dietary fat, fruit, and vegetable consumption: A best-evidence synthesis. *J Am Diet Assoc* 106(9):1434–1444.

Wu, J.Y., W.Y. Leung, et al. (2006). Effectiveness of telephone counselling by a pharmacist in reducing mortality in patients receiving polypharmacy: Randomised controlled trial. *Bmj* 333(7567):522.

BRIEF INTERVENTIONS IN PROMOTING
HEALTH BEHAVIOR CHANGE

CHAPTER 6

IMPLEMENTATION OF HEALTH BEHAVIOR CHANGE PRINCIPLES IN DENTAL PRACTICE

Jean Suvan, Angela Fundak, and Nina Gobat

Key Points of This Chapter

- The environment of oral care delivery has unique challenges and opportunities when promoting health behavior change.
- The patient activation model for the dental visit represents interwoven strands of the visit structure with techniques that can promote behavior change.
- Implementation complements, rather than complicates, the existing structure of the oral care appointment.

INTRODUCTION

The previous chapters of this book have described various elements of health behavior change from both the theoretical and practical perspective. Comparisons have been presented highlighting that health behavior change is not so dissimilar from our encounters with change in everyday life. As much as knowledge and understanding may have been increased or solidified as a result of reading the previous chapters, taking this information further into everyday practice may require some additional steps. This chapter will focus on some of the practical elements to consider as you continue to incorporate health behavior change approaches into your clinical practice.

Changing clinical practice carries some unique challenges. Recognition of this has, in turn, stimulated research in the area to provide further guidance on managing change in clinical work settings. Change management theory suggests that successful transformation is a result of the interaction between the *content of change* (objectives), the *context of change* (environment), and the *process of change* (implementation plan), and incorporates identification of barriers as a key element contributing to successful change (Dawes 1999; Pettigrew et al. 1989). In this chapter, the implementation of behavior change principles in the dental practice will be discussed within this framework of headings: content (objectives), context (environment), process (implementation plan), and barriers.

Most clinicians will be aware that the promotion of health behavior changes with the patients in their care may provide a range of benefits—increased success of treatment outcomes, decreased incidence of disease, increased confidence for both patient and clinician. Increasingly, as a growing percentage of the population are diagnosed with health decline that is often associated with "lifestyle" behaviors, the health professional is often required to have a dual focus—control of current disease while facilitating continuous self-management as part of an effective long-term solution. Oral health professionals are not exempt from this approach to patient care as we continue our efforts to manage disease and support health behavior change. The move from treating the disease (extraction, restoration, and gingivectomy) to minimally invasive dentistry and core preventive modalities reflects the impact of the growing change of focus in oral health care. More and more, we understand that regular, effective oral hygiene measures, cessation of tobacco use, management of alcohol consumption, and dietary control can contribute significantly to the reduction of risk for the development of diseases such as dental caries, periodontal disease, and oral cancer (Ramseier 2005). All of these elements may be within the capabilities of a positive union of professional support and continuous self-management by the patient.

The clinical encounter provides an opportunity for clinicians to develop a supportive, professional relationship that engages the patient in a dialogue about possible changes in health behaviors. This opportunity is often under-utilized. While some clinicians may find that applying health behavior change strategies or approaches is easy and natural, for others it may be more difficult. They may be more comfortable with the "traditional" role of the health professional as the expert provider of knowledge and advice to the patient. Indeed, the patient may also be accustomed to the role of "being told what to do" without complete understanding of why or indeed how to achieve the expectations of the clinician. Herein lies the dilemma in the clinician-patient relationship as they work together toward improved health and reduced disease—how can they understand each other? This chapter aims to provide a discussion framework for further exploration with your patients as you work together to develop an optimal plan of care for improved oral health.

> The environment of oral care delivery has unique challenges and opportunities when promoting health behavior change.

Content of change (the objectives)

If you encounter only patients with very low plaque scores, without periodontal disease, without caries, non-smokers, of normal weight, then you probably need not read further other than for sheer curiosity. However, many clinicians are often presented with care scenarios that reflect a plethora of multi-layered considerations from both a physiological (biological) and psychological (behavior) aspect. Both of these elements impact substantially on the adaptation required to maximize an effective communication pathway that may lead to supporting behavioral change. For experienced and inexperienced clinicians alike, the following examples are all too familiar:

> The woman who attends for continuous restorative dental care proclaiming that, "My mother had bad teeth, so I guess I have her genes."

> The man who comes to the practice for his maintenance visit presenting yet again with poor oral hygiene and the resulting consequences but this time comes with the demand for dental implants, as his friend has just received them.

> The patient who validates his lack of self-management by stating, "If I just come to see you regularly then everything will be okay."

Clinicians are often bewildered that some patients seem so motivated and compliant while others seem less than motivated or even non-responsive in spite of the same messages being delivered with somewhat the same enthusiasm in all situations. They may find themselves influenced by previous successes, applying solutions that worked with some patients when advising other patients. With persistence, using trial and error strategies, sooner or later many patients make lifestyle or self-care changes according to clinician recommendations. This could be due to the rapport that develops over time between the clinician and patient. In many cases, change is influenced by factors outside of the dental environment such as family, friends, media reports, or as a result of a series of other lifestyle changes. Just as common dental diseases are often multi-factorial in nature, change is often a cumulative process that builds a reasonable argument that can be accepted by the patient. If that argument is skillfully drawn from the patient as his or her own idea, then the reasons to change become more attractive. Therefore, if any of your patients could benefit from changes in self-care behaviors, the next step may be to consider how you feel about attempting to enhance your impact on the process.

Context of change (the environment)

When considering implementation of behavior change approaches, the context or environment is characterized by many elements, from attitudes, perceptions, past events, and current events to simply the physical space that you work in. It is important not to limit or underestimate the number of factors and their influence. Two particular factors related to perception are worthy of mention as we progress to consider context further.

Self-perception of our role as an oral health professional plays an important part in taking new steps to "activate" our patients. Traditionally, we may have been clinicians rendering technical procedures as interventions for disease treatment. Therefore, once a disease was defined, a treatment paradigm resulted thereafter. More recent knowledge of the chronic nature of diseases and multiple factors affecting them has brought focus on prevention and wellness. This knowledge has put disease management into a broader context. In recent times, we have seen that health professionals function in a much broader role as we think about health behavior change. In essence, clinicians may function as a type of "health coach" for chronic condition self-management in addition to providing treatment.

With easy access to a vast supply of information forms via the internet, many of our patients are increasingly independent in their health understanding, thoughts, and goals. As a result, the perspective of patients should always be considered a key element in the development of an ongoing plan of care. What is their perceived treatment need? Is it the same as their actual treatment needs? Understanding our patients' perspective of disease and health or their perception of our role is vital to our approach in conversing with them. Are they expecting us to "fix" or "cure"? Are they aware that much of dental care today is targeted toward prevention or complex disease management? The alignment of the clinician and patient in regard to the context of health care goals is paramount to supporting positive outcomes.

Process of change (the implementation plan)

You may be in a situation with extensive schedule flexibility, allowing you to spend lengthy amounts of time in discussion with your patients, or alternatively you may be bound to tight schedules with brief amounts of time. Regardless of the length of the visit, successful interactions are realistic. Remember the key lies in the approach.

There are many different ways to implement and integrate the approaches outlined in the previous chapters into daily practice. Implementation will depend on a variety of factors, most of which you will be the best person to identify. Above all, it is important to remember that behavior change strategies are designed to make your life easier. Approaches to the exploration of a patient's health behaviors can be a valuable learning experience for all. By exploring all the options for behavior change, the clinician and patient may discover new, effective solutions to concerns that were once regarded as unmanageable. In turn, the successes of each approach will increase confidence to address other issues or concerns for the patient and clinician. The wise proverb of "Success breeds success" is highly applicable to the field of improving oral health through behavior change.

Conversely, without exploration and understanding of the patient's intrinsic sense of change, the clinician often becomes bound to the "one-way traffic" conversation of advising and sometimes scolding. To repeat the same instructions can be frustrating for patient and clinician alike. It is akin to the definition of insanity; namely, doing the same thing and expecting a different result. In addition, this frustration may lead to resentment that can damage further relationship development. Herein lies the challenge of engagement toward success that is meaningful for the clinician and patient.

In reviewing the dental professional's content, context, and process for making even the smallest change in his or her own techniques or approaches, it is helpful to consider a perspective of the micro-environment, that is, the dental visit with an individual patient, and the macro-environment, referring to the overall practice setting or ethos.

MICRO-ENVIRONMENT: THE DENTAL VISIT

Easier than you think

> The patient activation model for the dental visit represents interwoven strands of the visit structure with techniques that can promote behavior change.

As we consider the scenarios at the beginning of this chapter, the question of where to start re-emerges. By focusing on a simple strategy based on the key underlying principles presented in the previous chapters, getting started can be easier than you think.

Use of a model designed specifically to guide dental clinicians in the exploration of integrating behavior change principles into everyday practice is presented for discussion (see Figure 6.1). The model depicts the "fabric" of the average health behavior change–focused dental visit. This fabric represents interwoven strands of the visit structure with techniques that can promote behavior change.

Patient activation fabric for the dental visit (implementation model)

The clinical dental visit is multi-layered and multi-functional. This model attempts to capture the interdependent elements of the visit using the concept of interwoven threads. Communication and information exchange blend together with clinical assessment and treatment. Thus, the success of the resulting "fabric" of the care plan is dependent on the interwoven strength of each thread (Figure 6.1).

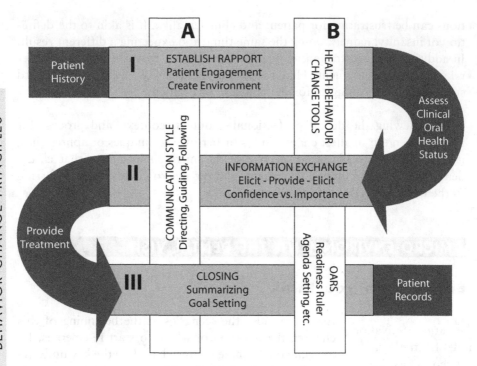

Figure 6.1. Patient activation fabric for the dental visit (implementation model).

The horizontal bands depict the three core strands of conversations constituting the visit. These bands transition directly into the curves, representing the clinical assessment or treatment that takes place between the conversations as part of the flow of the appointment. The bands are woven together through the vertical ribbons that signify the specific elements of the communication and interaction characterizing the approach. These vertical ribbons are consistent, yet flexible, recurring throughout the fabric, ready to provide stability as the horizontal bands are maneuvered around at each dental visit. The patient history and patient's records positioned at the start and end depict the critical elements of documentation that serve to weave one visit into the next.

Band I: Establish rapport

This is the opening part of the appointment. The goal is to quickly engage the patient and establish an open rapport. Accomplishing this depends on approach much more than the amount of time taken. A warm, courteous greeting is a critical start in creating an environment of mutual trust and respect. Ensuring that this initial greeting includes eye contact at the same level (i.e., both standing or both seated, and not when the patient is supine) will further support a comfortable environment. These simple actions create the perception of the patient and clinician having equal control of the situation rather than one being dominant. Having a sense of control can generate significant confidence, as the patient feels he or she has a valid role in the process of the appointment. This feeling of autonomy and confident collaboration, rather than passive observation, can greatly assist in patient activation that engages intrinsic motivation.

Implementation complements, rather than complicates, the existing structure of the oral care appointment.

Beginning with an open question that seeks the patient's prime concern or reason for attending the visit is another simple and valuable step. These opening moments set the scene for the remainder of the visit and can save you valuable time later in the session. For example, starting with the patient's concerns can allow you to detect potentially relevant clinical signs to inform your assessment. In addition, paying attention to this step communicates to your patient that you are interested in him or her as a person, making it easier at later stages of the visit to initiate brief conversations about change.

Before proceeding with the clinical assessment, it is important to briefly list the elements of the procedure to patients, then ask them if they would be happy for you to proceed with it at that time. Asking permission is a simple way to engage the patient while simultaneously encouraging a sense of autonomy. It may be helpful to explain to the patient the relevance of the information that he or she may hear you give to your assistant. These small actions help to keep your patient engaged in the consultation, rather than allowing the patient to shift to a passive role of lying helplessly throughout the assessment procedure. For example, before an assessment of probing pocket depth, the clinician may ask the patient what he or she knows about the range of measurements. The clinician can go on to clarify to the patient the range of measurements considered to be in "health." When the patient hears the clinician reporting any probing depths beyond the healthy range, he or she may understand that there is a potential breakdown of health. This can generate a valuable discussion, after the assessment, initiated by the patient with regard to periodontal health. Using this approach, the patient is actively asking for information. This may then lead to further requests for information or advice on self-care strategies for home.

Band II: Information exchange

This second band or portion of the interaction between clinician and patient would most often take place following initial clinical assessment of the patient's oral health status. It is likely the primary time for informing, although both you and your patient will seek and provide information throughout the visit. This exchange allows both parties to understand the other's perspective and create a more accurate picture of the clinical problem and approaches to effective management. This discussion can take many different forms. Through the lens of more traditional models, the practitioner may take an "expert" role, asking a series of closed clinical questions, which the patient is required to answer. The limitations of this approach have been discussed elsewhere in this book. Most noteworthy, however, is the effect this has on reinforcing passivity in the patient.

An alternative approach to providing information is one in which the practitioner maintains a focus on patient engagement. A valuable point in thinking about ways to do this is to remember that when talking to your patient, you are talking to an expert! No one knows his or her disease and life context better than the patient him- or herself. A simple framework for information exchange has been suggested to help you introduce new information in a guiding style of communication (Rollnick et al. 2007). The framework, discussed in chapters 3 and 4, can be easily remembered as "elicit-provide-elicit." Starting with what the patient already knows (elicit) immediately encourages patients to think, reflect, and acknowledge their own expertise. From that starting point you can then—with permission—tailor the information you offer to patients (provide). Perhaps the most important step is the question that follows, exploring what sense the patient makes of information provided (elicit). This question can open the door to dialogue rich with opportunity for discussions about change.

Not all exchanges of information will happen in the guiding style of communication. As described in chapter 3, skillful communication involves flexibly shifting between styles. Remember that the communication styles are characterized by the attitude the practitioner takes. We suggest that when talking about behavior change it is useful to engage the expertise of the patient and to use a guiding style. Elicit-provide-elicit can be a helpful framework to help you shift into this style. However, there may well be other times—for example, when you are giving feedback about your clinical examination—when you may choose to use the directing style of communication. To do this skillfully, it should be (1) personally relevant, (2) clearly stated, and (3) well timed (Rollnick et al. 2007).

Leading into and moving on from this middle phase of the visit, you may be performing a number of clinical tasks including assessment and treatment. Conversations about behavior change are most valuable when you and your patient are able to speak freely. Be mindful not to have these conversations when your patient is unable to be an equal participant, such as when the patient is physically incapable of speaking or may be feeling pain or discomfort during or after clinical procedures. Therefore, once any procedure has been commenced, your talking should be limited to checking for patient comfort or confirming agreement to continue with further steps of the procedure.

Band III: Closing

The third band takes place and functions as a closing to the visit. It may involve a brief summary of the clinical treatment that has been provided together with any expected side effects or post-treatment discomfort. Equally as important is that it serves to briefly summarize behavior change discussions. It provides the clinician with the opportunity to review the agreed goals or plan of action suggested by the patient in Band II. To ensure this is collaborative, the clinician should ask the patient if there is anything he or she would like to add to the plan and check that the most important points have been covered. Further treatment options may also be discussed if the patient is not too tired. However, this is not typically the best time for most patients to discuss important facts, as they are usually focused on leaving the dental chair as soon as the appointment has concluded.

Ribbon A: Communication style

In the previous chapters, styles of communication were presented, highlighting that a spectrum exists with directing and following at opposite extremes and guiding in the middle as an intermediary style engaging both parties equally. A skillful movement between the three styles constitutes the well-managed interaction with the patient. In the model, communication style is labelled as a vertical ribbon interwoven through the entire visit. This portrays that at certain times during the visit, a particular style will tend to be more advantageous than the others. Maximum patient engagement without compromising the clinician's responsibility and ability to provide important information will be facilitated through use of a guiding style. Fundamental communication techniques such as asking open questions can encourage the two-way communication that characterizes a guiding style. However, this does not infer that it is the only style of communication used during the visit.

Throughout all communication interactions with the patient, it is valuable to remember that asking questions should only occur when the patient is able to respond comfortably (i.e., without interference from instruments and/or the clinician). Without this consideration, communication success will be challenged, as the patient may feel a loss of control.

Ribbon B: Health behavior change tools

The second vertical ribbon in the model is comprised of the many behavior change tools highlighted throughout the previous chapters to facilitate patient activation or interaction throughout the visit. Like Ribbon A, each clinician may choose the tool he or she feels will be most beneficial at certain points in the visit or conversation. The choice is driven by the goal to provide a relaxed atmosphere where conversations can be spontaneous and individualized to each patient. Some of these tools include agenda setting, the readiness ruler, the typical day strategy, open questions, affirmation, reflective listening, summarizing, or expressing empathy.

"Your patient is here"

As we review the everyday routine, remember that integrating aspects of behavior change into the dental visit can be a smooth process that adds value to patient care and clinician satisfaction. Rather than replacing the framework of the dental visit, the tools and principles weave into your everyday activities, creating opportunities for small conversations that can make a big difference in the quality of care you deliver. The patient scenarios that follow are based on the model of the dental visit presented. They are intended to illustrate or analyze examples of a dental visit using communication styles and behavior change tools to enhance patient engagement and promote positive health behavior changes. Short comments to the right of the dialogue help to clarify these elements.

In designing the scenario that follows, we have chosen to highlight certain clinical presentations and settings. In addition, some of the more "unspoken" elements of the dental visit, such as the feelings or perceptions of the patient and clinician, body language, and visit flow, are described. In this way we hope to give you some illustration of how this may translate into everyday clinical practice. Of course, we cannot illustrate every possible clinical scenario that you may encounter. All patients are individual and unique. We encourage you to think about how these principles are illustrated in the examples and to draw some parallels to your own daily clinical practice. You will recognize many steps or approaches that you may already use regularly in practice. Others may be less familiar. The goal is to enhance your use of these approaches to maximize your impact with the least amount of effort.

Single behavior patient scenario

The setting:

- a general dental practice;

- 45-minute 4-month periodontal maintenance appointment;

- the clinician has not seen this patient previously, although he has been a patient in the practice for some time.

  Prior to the visit:

- the clinician reviews the patient records, checking for patient history in terms of clinical status, patient concerns, and previous clinician recommendations;

- the clinician notes that, at the last visit, the patient's plaque and gingival inflammation levels had increased from previous and that oral hygiene was discussed.

  The key clinical presentation features for this 45-year-old male patient at the prior visit were:

- generalized (progressive) moderate periodontitis;

- Grade II mobility of the maxillary incisors;

- localized gingival recession;

- bleeding score 46%;

- plaque score 78%;

- no relevant medical history.

The key behavioral presentation features for this patient were:

- irregular brushing and interproximal cleaning habits;

- dietary management is good;

- non-smoker;

- professional dental care is regular (three times per year);

- time management demands are high.

Band I: Establishing rapport

A member of the practice team has seated the patient in the dental chair. The clinician walks into the treatment room, sits down, makes eye contact with the patient, and greets him sincerely. *Body language is key here.*

Clinician: "Good morning Mr. R. I don't think that we have met before, have we?"	*Warm introductory greeting* *Shakes hands with patient*
Patient: "No, I usually see Jenny, who looks after my teeth. But I was told that I would be seeing you today."	
Clinician: "Oh good! Well, my name is Serena and it is a pleasure to meet you. I have reviewed all of the records we have on your care to date. How have you been since your last visit to the practice?"	*Open question*
Patient: "Oh, as busy as ever, you know there are never enough hours in the day trying to manage the business and keep everyone happy. Plus we have just moved so everything is really chaotic!"	
Clinician: "It sounds like you keep a hectic pace with many things to balance at one time. How have things been surviving in the 'tooth and gum department'?"	*Reflective listening statement* *Open question*
Patient: "Well, you know, I try my best but I don't always have the time to really pay much attention."	

Clinician: "You try to do the best you can with the time available. What concerns do you have that I could help you with today?"

Reflective listening statement
Open question— agenda setting (eliciting patient concerns)

Patient: "Well, I don't like the color of my teeth and I get bleeding occasionally when I brush or if I remember to floss! Sometimes, the gum areas get sore so I brush them a bit more often and that seems to clear it up. I know that my gums are not as good as they should be. Jenny tells me the same thing every time!"

Clinician: "So you're worried about discoloration and some bleeding during cleaning. Anything else?"

Reflective listening statement
Open question— agenda setting (checking re: patient's list of concerns)

Patient: "Well, I've decided I would like to have these middle two teeth replaced with implants. My friend just had some put in. They are really great. He says they don't even need cleaning, just always look great. That would make my life easier. Less of the scraping that makes my mouth hurt after I come here. No offense but it is so unpleasant. You know that stain that always comes on my front teeth really bothers me and I think the gap in the middle might be getting wider. Implants could solve the whole story."

Clinician: "You'd also like us to consider some solutions to the discoloration of your teeth today and maybe talk about implants. Anything else?"

Reflective listening statement
Resisting the righting reflex
Open question— continues with agenda setting

Patient: "No, that's it."

Clinician: "OK, so I don't really have any specific concerns to add to that list. Perhaps I could to take a look at your teeth and gums, and we can then discuss those concerns in a bit more detail?"

Completes agenda setting
Asking permission

Patient: "Sure."

Band I commentary

In these brief moments, the clinician has enhanced the environment for positive behavior change by using some simple techniques:

1. Maintaining equal status position

   Greeting the patient in a position at the same level (in this case sitting) maintains the perception of equal status. When the patient is seated in the dental chair and the clinician is standing, this automatically places the clinician at a height advantage that may be interpreted as a superior position.

2. Agenda setting

   The clinician sets an agenda with the patient by asking a series of open questions to elicit his questions and concerns. The agenda setting strategy consists of both open questioning and reflective listening statements. The clinician is solely focused on understanding how the patent hopes to be helped during the consultation. At the same time, this allows her to build rapport with the patient and engage his expertise.

   Note how the practitioner avoids jumping in to address any of these concerns too early in the consultation. Instead she maintains a mental "step back," simply taking note of the patient's agenda. Doing this allows the clinician to plan how best to use her time, as well as to start her clinical assessment and to get an understanding of what the patient expects as an outcome of the consultation.

3. Resisting the righting reflex

   Notice how the practitioner avoids addressing the patient's request for implants directly. Instead she reframes this request as an item on the patient's agenda, that is, "solutions to the discoloration."

4. Asking permission

   The clinician reinforces the patient's autonomy by asking permission to proceed with the exam. It is unlikely that a patient will say no at this point. After all, patients expect a clinical examination when they come for their appointments! Asking permission communicates respect for the patient's right to choose and engages the patient more fully in the clinical exam, which is often a passivity-inducing procedure.

Assess clinical oral health status

The clinician completes the oral assessment consisting of inspection of the various soft and hard tissues. The clinical status has not improved over his last visit in spite of re-instruction of oral hygiene techniques that was noted from the last visit. It is now possible to compare the patient's concerns with those of the clinician. The clinician instantly and automatically has the goal for the visit in mind.

1. Current patient concern

    At this particular visit, Mr. R has come with the wish to arrange a plan to have dental implants to replace his two maxillary incisors. His friend has recently received an implant and is very happy with the results. He sees this as a solution to his discolored and migrating anterior teeth.

2. Current clinician concerns

    The clinician's view is that the patient's oral hygiene is the problem to be addressed. Implants are not feasible at this time. It would be inappropriate to place them in an oral environment with high plaque levels and the subsequent levels of gingival inflammation and recurring increase in periodontal probing depths.

3. Health behavior of concern

    The health behavior of concern for this patient is his oral hygiene self-care routine.

4. Goal of the visit

    The goal is then to motivate him to improve his self-care so that the implants might eventually be feasible to consider as a possible solution for the anterior incisor mobility. However, remember the patient would like a solution for the appearance of his front teeth. The challenge still remains to unify the goals.

Band II information exchange

The patient is returned to an upright position following the clinical assessment to continue the interaction with the clinician. Notice that it has only been possible to understand both the patient concerns and the clinician concerns following an initial oral assessment. Resisting the temptation to provide

IMPLEMENTATION OF HEALTH BEHAVIOR CHANGE PRINCIPLES

information to the patient prior to the oral assessment allows the clinician to reinforce an individual patient-centered approach. Even if information to be provided is relatively generic, a brief view of the mouth, together with eliciting views from the patient, allows the clinician to customize delivery of the information. This is done within the focus of the patient's concern to synchronize his goals.

Clinician: "OK, thanks for your patience while we reviewed how everything looks today."	
Patient: "No problem. I was a bit concerned to hear that some of those numbers were bigger than the "healthy" range you mentioned before you started."	
Clinician: "Yes, you are right. Some of the gum pocket measurements are deeper than we would like to see. Would it be OK for us to spend the next few minutes talking about those concerns?"	*Raises the topic* *Asks permission*
Patient: "Yeah, great."	
Clinician: "What do you think is going on there?"	*Open question (elicits what the patient already knows)*
Patient: "Well, I've been told before that if you don't brush properly your gums can start to pull away from your teeth. So I guess that's what could be happening to me."	
Clinician: "Yes, you are right. The gum attachment can become less secure around the teeth when bacteria are continuously causing inflammation that you may notice as bleeding. What other kinds of things do you know about gum disease?"	*Open question (eliciting current knowledge)*
Patient: "Well, I've also heard that some people even have their teeth taken out because of gum disease that gets into the jawbone."	
Clinician: "Yes, that happens to some people. Can I review some information with you about that?"	*Asks permission to provide information*

Patient: "Sure."

Clinician: "Periodontitis is a progressive disease. What I mean by that is that if left to its' own devices the disease will keep attacking the gums and then move into the bones and so on. The teeth may even start to move slightly due to the inflammation and reduced bone support. This inflammation can develop around implants just the same as around the teeth. Fortunately there are ways of slowing or controlling this process. Some of the things you've no doubt heard about ..."   *Provides information*

Patient: "Like flossing and coming to see you for some scraping or 'gum gardening' as Jenny jokingly calls it."

Clinician: "Exactly. Doing those things like flossing, regular brushing with a good technique, and coming to appointments like these—we refer to all of that as 'self-care.' So, doing all those things regularly can really help slow the progress of the disease. What sense do you make of all this?"   *Elicits response to the information provided*

Patient: "Well, I was just thinking, you know ... my uncle had this when he was quite young. That kind of worries me. Is there much chance for me?"

Clinician: "That's a difficult question to answer. Like I said, there are things we can look at to help slow down the progression of the disease. So, in some ways how it progresses is really up to you. I'd like to understand a bit more about how important this is to you right now. Can I ask you a couple of questions?"   *Introduces readiness ruler*   *Asks permission*

Patient: "Sure."

Clinician: "If you were to rate the importance of self-care of on a scale of 1 to 10, with 1 being not important and 10 being very important, where would you say you are today?"   *Practitioner asks a scaling question on importance*

Patient: "Definitely a 10! I don't want to lose my teeth and if I do, I want those implants."   *Change talk*

Clinician: "So it is very important for you to keep your gums as healthy as possible. If we look at how confident you feel about regularly following your self-care routine, where would you rate yourself today on that 1 to 10 scale?"	*Reflective listening* *Practitioner moves on to ask about confidence*
Patient: "Well, I would have to say about a 4 because I try to do better but I just don't have the time to do everything."	*Change talk*
Clinician: "OK, so although time is an issue, you do try to make an effort with your self-care routine. You scored yourself at a 4, why a 4 and not, say, a 2 or a 3?"	
Patient: "Well I do manage to do the full routine some days. And I actually feel quite pleased with myself on those days, you know."	*Change talk follows*
Clinician: "You give yourself a pat on the back."	*Reflective listening statement*
Patient: "Yeah, I do. I have a really busy life, you know, and so it really takes an effort to fit in my cleaning routine."	
Clinician: "And there are days that you manage this."	*Practitioner focuses on the patient's abilities*
Patient: "Exactly."	
Clinician: "Tell me a bit more about those days."	*Asks for elaboration*
Patient: "Well, sometimes it's because my gums have been bleeding a bit more than usual and I know that it's because I've not been so good at keeping up with my routine. And then when I get back into it, I can't imagine why I don't do it. The bleeding stops and I actually feel much better about myself."	*Change talk*
Clinician: "You really notice a difference in the condition of your gums and how you feel about yourself when you clean regularly. So, what might help with shifting your confidence up a notch, say from a 4 to a 5?"	*Reflective listening statement* *Readiness ruler question*

> Patient: "Well, I just have to do it. And maybe not give myself such a hard time about not doing it. Because sometimes I just think, oh, what's the use? I'll just skip it tonight. But maybe it's just about giving it a go and doing something. That's better than nothing, right?"
>
> *Patient is defining a plan for himself*
> *Change talk*
>
> Clinician: "Sure, because this is important to you. You've said that and you know that, so even the smallest effort is something. And it really is up to you."
>
> *Reflective listening statement*
> *Autonomy support*
>
> Patient: "Well, I don't want to end up like my uncle ... and I do wish they looked better."
>
> *Change talk*
>
> Clinician: "So, it sounds like you would like to give it another go. I can plan to evaluate things again in 3 months. Sound okay?"
>
> Patient: "Sure. Sounds reasonable."

Band II commentary

Notice the difference in the concerns of the patient and those of the clinician. The challenge of this band is to merge the two and to facilitate identification by the patient of the need for improved oral hygiene. The clinician has tailored the communication to maximize the opportunity for behavior change using further behavior change tools.

1. Raising the topic

   Raising a topic of behavior change may fall naturally out of the clinical examination. In this example, the patient had spoken of his worries about the condition of his gums. Clinical examination revealed that there were clinical indicators of deterioration. This observation, together with the patient's pre-stated agenda item, opened the door quite naturally to a conversation about self-care. Keeping watch for these opportunities and steering the conversation toward behavior change is one way you can start to integrate these ideas into your everyday practice.

   Once again, asking permission to speak about a topic demonstrates respect for the patient's right to choose and fosters a collaborative conversational atmosphere. Patients seldom refuse an invitation to talk about something even if they feel a bit reluctant to address the topic. Raising a topic without asking permission can leave a patient feeling defensive and can create avoidable resistance.

IMPLEMENTATION OF HEALTH
BEHAVIOR CHANGE PRINCIPLES

2. Elicit-provide-elicit

In this example, the clinician sees an opportunity for giving the patient some information about periodontitis by using a guiding style of communication. She uses the "elicit-provide-elicit" (E-P-E) framework described earlier in this chapter and in chapters 3 and 4. Notice the patient's responses to her questioning at each stage of the E-P-E strategy. Providing information in this way encourages patients to reflect and think about what meaning it may have to them personally. Here the patient speaks about a family member who also experienced periodontal disease. The information provided by the clinician takes the form of a dialogue between the two parties and the patient spontaneously raises questions himself.

A patient who is actively engaged in a consultation will naturally ask questions. This is when patients are most receptive to receiving information and processing it in a meaningful way. Sharing clinical information in this way makes it immediately relevant and personally meaningful to the patient.

3. Readiness ruler

There are no set rules about when to use which strategy. In this example, we illustrate the use of a readiness ruler following the E-P-E strategy. Notice how the clinician uses the strategy in relation to a specific and clearly stated behavior change, that is, self-care. A common mistake in attempting to use this strategy occurs when practitioners don't identify the change focus clearly. In this example, the clinician understands that self-care is really important for this patient, and that the patient has low confidence in being able to do this regularly. By asking curious, structured open questions, in a guiding style of communication, she is able to elicit the seeds of a change plan from this patient. "Ask RIC" (Readiness = Importance + Confidence) is an easy acronym to remember for integrating this component in the approach to behavior change.

Notice, too, how the readiness ruler is a *conversational device*. It is used to facilitate talk about change. Change is not a linear process—it is unlikely that you will observe incremental increase in readiness across sessions for your patients. So the numbers that patients give you when you are using this strategy tell you little in and of themselves. The skill of using this strategy lies in how you use the numbers to engage the patient in talking about his or her motivations.

Further information on the use of a readiness ruler, together with other illustrations of this in clinical practice, are provided in chapters 4 and 5.

4. Change talk

As discussed in previous chapters in this text, the goal of approaches to behavior change is for the patient to present his or her own arguments for change. You will hear this in a patient's expression of change talk. Notice how the clinician structures her conversation to elicit change talk. In this interchange, the patient begins to describe a plan for change that makes sense to him and that emerges from his own motivations.

Provide clinical treatment

The clinician continues with the visit, proceeding to render the treatment that is a part of the maintenance appointment.

Band III closing

The patient is again returned to an upright position in the chair following completion of the treatment procedures. Often you will hear a patient breathe a sigh of relief, as it may be the first chance for a full intake of air since the treatment began! Clinicians are sometimes forgetful that breathing freely is often difficult for the patient throughout the treatment phase of an appointment. When the patient is finally able to close his or her mouth, happy that the procedures are finished, the next thing he or she would really like to do is leave the chair. Unfortunately, some clinicians feel that this a good time for continued discussion. Being sensitive to the patient's body language and verbal responses can help the clinician decide on an appropriate close to the appointment.

The clinician has removed her mask and gloves, returning to a sitting position to re-establish eye contact with the patient to close the appointment.

Clinician: "We have talked about a number of items   *Summarizes*
today. Let's see if I can summarize what we've been
talking about so far. Because the health of your gums is
important to you, you are going to go on with your
routine even if you miss now and then. You are just
going to keep going even if only a small amount is
possible. We have agreed to re-evaluate this at your next
visit. We could also discuss the value and feasibility of
implants for you at that time. Anything I've left out?
Anything you would like to ask before you go?"
Patient: "I think that is about covered for now. I'll make
my next appointment and we'll see how the gums are
then."

Band III commentary

Notice the clear transition to, and intent of, this phase of the visit. The focus here is to summarize key elements of the appointment and to clarify the agreed plan in a concise and positive manner. In addition, the goal is to end with a thread that can easily be picked up at the beginning of the next visit. Key techniques aid this in a few brief moments.

1. Summarizing

   Notice how the practitioner ties the various strands of the consultation together in a single summary statement. To confirm with the patient that the summary statement captures his understanding of the visit reinforces collaboration.

Multiple behavior patient scenario

At times, patients may present with more than one health behavior to be considered. This can perpetuate a further layer of complexity in conversing with patients about steps toward health behavior change. Imagine Mr. R, our previously described patient. He arrives today with poor oral hygiene, and he has had a very busy time recently so has returned to his smoking. In addition, he has a number of sites of recurrent caries that the clinician suspects may be sugar intake related. In this type of scenario, the dental visit follows a similar sequence, with many of the behavior change tools being applicable in the same manner as described in the single behavior scenario. However, there is one major difference. This is the challenge presented due to the multiple behaviors to address. If all are discussed in one visit, there is a risk of information overload. In addition, the patient may not be equally ready to discuss each of the behaviors. There may be negative feelings associated with some and not others. If you "start off on the wrong foot" you may provoke resistance, then minimizing your opportunity to engage the patient or have even the smallest influence on any of the behaviors.

As mentioned in some of the previous chapters, agenda setting is a useful strategy to consider when there are several behavior changes that you may like to talk with a patient about. There are a variety of ways to do this, but the key element of using this strategy is to take a "mental step back" and provide a brief overview of the different topics that can be discussed. Consider the following piece of dialogue. By setting an agenda, the practitioner opens the door to a conversation about change in which the patient is a willing participant.

In the previous case example, we illustrated the use of agenda setting at the start of the consultation. This piece of dialogue illustrates agenda setting during Band II, where the practitioner uses the strategy to agree on the focus of conversation. The following dialogue example could take place at any stage during Band II.

IMPLEMENTATION OF HEALTH BEHAVIOR CHANGE PRINCIPLES

Clinician: "Okay, thanks for your patience while we reviewed how everything looks today. From what you have already told me and from our review, it seems that you have a number of concerns."	
Patient: "Well, yes! I know my gums are not so healthy and smoking again is probably not a good idea."	*Patient raises multiple behaviors*
Clinician: "You are right. We often find with other patients that unhealthy gums and smoking are not good partners! We know that the gums can't resist bacteria as well if you are a smoker. So, I guess there are two aspects here to consider, bacteria around the gums and the impact of smoking."	*Practitioner clarifies potential behavior change topics*
Patient: (sighs) "Well, I just can't see myself getting free of the cigarettes right now, to be honest."	*Low readiness to change smoking*
Clinician: "Well, you're the one who knows what is possible now. How about other areas to think about?"	*Autonomy support*
Patient: "I could get back into my regular brushing routine now that I am finally in my own house permanently."	*Change talk*
Clinician: "So making some changes to your self-care routine seems more manageable right now. Perhaps we could spend a few moments talking about that?"	*Reflective listening statement* *Behavior change focus agreed* *Practitioner initiates talk about this behavior change*

IMPLEMENTATION OF HEALTH
BEHAVIOR CHANGE PRINCIPLES

Commentary

The clinician notices the potential to talk about a number of behavior change topics and sets an agenda with the patient. By "stepping back" and clarifying the different topics that can be discussed, she can agree on a focus for the discussion. Had the patient not raised the subject of smoking himself, the clinician could have done so at this stage, thereby raising a potentially awkward subject in a non-threatening manner. Talking about "other patients" helps normalize these discussions and externalizes the behaviors for discussion, minimizing potential for the patient to feel attacked or blamed.

Until now, we have discussed the principles presented in the context of the dental visit, that is, the setting of the clinician and the patient in the dental treatment room. However, this environment is not positioned in solitude but rather is part of the entire dental practice and the specific patients that will visit during any particular day. We will move on to discuss important elements of the dental practice in implementing health behavior change approaches.

MACRO-ENVIRONMENT: THE PRACTICE SETTING

Thinking back to the implications of the change management theory stated earlier in this chapter, the inference is that setting goals and aiming for a supportive environment (i.e., the practice setting) to formulate a plan could be paramount to successful implementation of behavior change approaches in practice. Consideration of a bottom-up approach vs. a top-down approach, thus giving the opportunity for involvement by all practice members, is more likely to facilitate change. In addition, identification of potential obstacles is an integral part of the plan formation. Utilization of a team approach may be vital to overcoming the barriers to effective behavioral change (Needleman et al. 2006).

Importance of support

The practice environment cannot be ignored when considering a change in how an individual practices or relates to patients. The patient interacts with a number of colleagues during the course of his or her visit in the dental practice. Ideally this interaction should be supportive of the promotion of any agreed behavior change between the patient and clinician. This aligned support can be of immeasurable value as the patient feels valued and aware that others understand. Conversely, if co-workers are insensitive or contradictory to the behavior change opportunities between clinician and patient, then motivation may be considerably decreased. For example, if the clinician and patient communication has included a discussion on the benefits of using a particular oral care product, this should be supported by the remainder of the dental team. Often patients will ask the practice manager/receptionist his or her opinion. This is where the macro- (practice) environment needs to be consistent. From this perspective, the clinician may also consider the value of behavior change skills within the context of promoting effective practice management. This approach may be helpful to create a practice environment that is supportive of positive behavior change for all involved in the pursuit of improved oral health care. The larger context of the practice is that many elements significantly influence clinician routines and approaches.

Overcoming potential obstacles to practice implementation

The term "obstacle" often carries a negative connotation. However, anticipation of obstacles can already go a long way to ensuring they do not exist. Much can be learned from evidence published on the integration of tobacco cessation counselling into a dental practice setting. It has been suggested that this involves a change in knowledge, attitudes, and behavior of the dental team members. Research findings from this field have suggested many possible deterrents to the required changes needed to facilitate behavior change interventions, including

- lack of feeling that it is an appropriate part of the clinician's responsibility,

- doubts by clinician and patient of the value or legitimacy of counselling,

- lack of team approach and communication,

- lack of early education,

- fear of damaging dentist-patient rapport, and

- failures in previous attempts.

Variability in potential barriers may be present and dependent on the various external and internal factors, such as population level cultural factors or dental practice organizational factors. The importance of well-designed "systems" and communication within the team has been highlighted in studies from the medical community (Braun et al. 2004). Although the barriers identified may be similar, the magnitude of each in a given setting at a set point in time may vary. This infers that each individual and practice must take the time to analyze the barriers relevant to their specific situation and appropriately set up a well-designed, step-by-step plan.

To facilitate required changes, the dental team members may need to expand not only their knowledge and skills but also their perception of roles (Mecklenburg 2001). The dental practice needs to include the involvement of dental auxiliaries in promoting behavior change recommendations such as tobacco use cessation programs (Monaghan 2002; Watt et al. 2004).

This team approach would include engagement of all practice co-workers in the formulation of the plan, therefore avoiding implementation that is haphazard or individual (Christen 2001). Formulation of a plan or ongoing communication once a plan has been implemented also serves to confirm or alleviate perceptions of barriers. For example, lack of time has been cited as a barrier to tobacco cessation counselling; however, many approaches based on brief intervention have been proposed suggesting that impact on schedule is minimal. Each team should assess the issue of time in the context of their setting.

Cultural beliefs can also affect attitudes toward oral health, specifically oral health behaviors and practices and use of available dental services. Oral health care providers have been reminded to be culturally sensitive when providing care for refugees and immigrants, as well as when producing health educating materials and in targeting approaches to oral health promotion and care delivery in multicultural societies (Hobdell et al. 2002).

The likelihood of health care clinicians pursuing meaningful efforts to assist patients with behavioral change is closely linked to clinicians' own beliefs regarding their efficacy in such roles. Such beliefs produce their effects by influencing how practitioners feel, think, and motivate themselves and are based on thoughtful consideration of previous accomplishments, observations of others in such roles, external encouragement, and one's own emotional investment in the process (Bandura 1997).

The process of receiving dental care is a very unique experience for many patients. The oral cavity is such a sensitive, personal, and emotionally charged area of the body, and many dental patients must develop a high level of trust in their clinician in order to be comfortable undergoing even routine dental care procedures. Therefore, once a compatible dental clinician is found, many patients maintain a strong personal allegiance. Clinicians also understand the sometimes "fragile" nature of the relationship and may tend to consciously avoid any activities or discussions with patients that they fear may threaten or disrupt the ongoing professional rapport.

Actual accomplishments or mastery experiences are the most influential sources of confidence because they are based on one's own beliefs about success—in other words, "nothing succeeds like success itself." In the same way, unfavorable outcomes that may occur prior to success can undermine future efforts. Learning to persist through discouraging times can help clinicians and patients feel more in control. When people become convinced that they have the ability to succeed, they not only persevere in the face of adversity, they also rebound more quickly from setbacks.

Verbal encouragement is also a potentially valuable source of confidence. When individuals are verbally persuaded that they have the capability to perform a given task, they are more likely to try harder to do what is asked of them. Although not as strong as successful performance or vicarious experiences, if positive feedback is within realistic bounds, it can encourage change (Newman 2006).

PRACTICAL GUIDANCE FOR BEGINNERS (OR NON-BEGINNERS)

As with any new skill or assimilation of new knowledge, practice makes perfect. The application of the principles that support health behavior change may seem challenging as you have been reading through this chapter and indeed this book! However, this discussion has been provided in "slow motion" to illustrate each step in the process as part of the learning experience. As each step is explored, both the clinician and patient will become more confident in utilizing these new approaches in relationship development. In addition, this confidence equates to increased speed in application during the appointment. During this transition, it is helpful to keep a checklist of handy reminders of the process as your confidence increases.

- Behavior change tools and strategies are designed to make life easier, not more stressful. Becoming skillful takes time and persistence.

- Change is a process, not an event. It takes time, intention, and effort for both your patient and for your own clinical practice.

- Imagine you are the patient—how would you like to be treated?

- Allow yourself to make mistakes.

- Your patients will be your greatest teachers—they provide immediate feedback on how you're doing through their moment-by-moment responses. Watch your patient's response!

- Don't be afraid of a few seconds of silence. Give your patients time to answer and take time as you need to form your own statements.

- Focus on discovering new things about the patient. And be prepared for surprises!

- Start small—start with one skill at a time, step by step (e.g., practice listening for 1 day/week, open questions for a day/week).

- Give yourself the best chance of success—don't pick your toughest patient when starting to practice this approach! Start with someone you have a good rapport with and go from there.

- A good guide follows a plan. Purposefully structuring your consultations can create opportunities for conversations about change.

- Practice listening by making short, frequent summaries of the essence of what your patient has been talking about.

- Remember behavior change is individual, so avoid leaping to conclusions or making judgments.

- Accept your limitations. Humility, modesty, and persistence create fertile ground for change.

- Respecting patient autonomy means accepting that some patients may choose not to change their behavior. This is not a failure. The only failure occurs when the engagement has not been attempted.

- Have fun with it!

SUMMARY

The relationship between clinician and patient within the dental setting provides a unique combination of elements that are not encountered in any other health care environment. The most challenging of these elements is the simple fact that caring for oral health involves the restriction of the fundamental means of communication—talking. As you provide treatment for the patient, you automatically remove an intrinsic source of power, comfort, and ability to feel in control. Without the opportunity to comfortably voice opinion or freely respond, the patient's perception of a positive relationship may be challenged. Therefore, as a dental clinician, you need to engage all your skills in establishing a positive relationship with your patient throughout the professional association in the micro- and macro-environments of the dental setting.

Fortunately, there are some simple core principles that can help you both to manage the impact of the dental setting and to seize opportunities to promote oral health. Throughout this chapter and the content of this book, frameworks for the application of these principles have been illustrated. However, just as each clinician's approach may vary, we understand that the patient response is also variable. This reflection of human nature provides a rich opportunity to create a successful partnership of care between you and your patient in exploring both diversity and commonality on the path to improved health. Taking the first step will move you forward to a great adventure!

REFERENCES

Bandura, A. (1997). *Self-Efficacy: The Exercise of Control.* New York: W.H. Freeman.

Braun, B.L., J.B. Fowles, et al. (2004). Smoking-related attitudes and clinical practices of medical personnel in Minnesota. *Am J Prev Med* 27(4):316–322.

Christen, A.G. (2001). Tobacco cessation, the dental profession, and the role of dental education. *J Dent Educ* 65(4):368–374.

Dawes, M. (1999). *Evidence-based practice, a primer for health care professionals.* Edinburgh: Churchill Livingstone.

Hobdell, M., J. Sinkford, et al. (2002). 5.2 Ethics, equity and global responsibilities in oral health and disease. *Eur J Dent Educ* 6 Suppl 3:167–178.

Mecklenburg, R.E. (2001). Tobacco prevention and control in dental practice: The future. *J Dent Educ* 65(4):375–384.

Monaghan, N. (2002). What is the role of dentists in smoking cessation? *Br Dent J* 193(11):611–612.

Needleman, I., S. Warnakulasuriya, et al. (2006). Evaluation of tobacco use cessation (TUC) counselling in the dental office. *Oral Health Prev Dent* 4(1):27–47.

Newman, A.M. (2006). Self-efficacy. In: I.M. Lubkin and P.D. Larsen, *Chronic Illness: Impact and Interventions*. Sudbury, MA: Jones and Bartlett, 105–120.

Pettigrew, A., L. McKee, et al. (1989). Managing strategic service change in the NHS. *Health Serv Manage Res* 2(1):20–31.

Ramseier, C.A. (2005). Potential impact of subject-based risk factor control on periodontitis. *J Clin Periodontol* 32 Suppl 6:283–290.

Rollnick, S., W.R. Miller, et al. (eds.). (2007). *Motivational Interviewing in Health Care*. New York: Guilford Press.

Watt, R., P. McGlone, et al. (2004). The facilitating factors and barriers influencing change in dental practice in a sample of English general dental practitioners. *Br Dent J* 197(8):485–489; discussion 475.

CHAPTER 7

HEALTH BEHAVIOR CHANGE EDUCATION

Philip S. Richards

Key Points of This Chapter

- The development and integration of behaviorally based dental care within the clinical education of students has not been substantial since the middle of the twentieth century.
- Patient self-management strategies and interactive methods to encourage informed patient choice are rapidly developing areas in health care. In order for such changes to be implemented in dental practice, changes in both the professional training and cultural norms in dental care will be needed.
- To provide an educational environment that will allow students to independently provide behavior change strategies in the practice of dentistry, a specific curriculum must be created and implemented to encourage such strategies.
- In general, for health behavior change curricula, a knowledge base attained through lectures, Problem-Based Learning, or E-Learning and clinical skills attained through clinical instructions and practices are required.
- Assessment universally drives the process of learning. Whatever the circumstances, all educators must focus on what the graduate needs for optimum performance and lifelong self-development through active learning, while being accountable to the society they must serve as ethical clinicians.

INTRODUCTION

As outlined in the previous chapters, motivating patients regarding behaviors associated with health and disease is a central part of the practice of all health professionals. From an educational point of view, these activities are supposed to be based on theoretical knowledge, evidence from research, and interactive skills learned and practiced during professional training.

Behavior change interventions for patients may be delivered during active treatments by health care providers as well as separate educational programs targeted at risk populations in communities (Redman 2007). The need for further health behavior content in the education of health professionals, particularly in medicine and dentistry, has been well documented. The ability of the oral health care team to successfully guide behavioral change in patients is one of the most important factors for long-term oral health maintenance in the population. Health professionals' perceptions of their patients, communication with patients, and effective models of professional interaction were identified more than 50 years ago as critically relevant to professional practice and thus appropriate targets for education (Gochman 1997).

HISTORY OF MEDICAL AND DENTAL EDUCATION

In medicine

Hundreds of years ago, societies began systematically caring for their citizens by promoting their health and welfare. Early in the twentieth century, the Carnegie Foundation for the Advancement of Teaching funded a series of reports on professional education in the United States. The fourth report, Abraham Flexner's 1910 study of medical education, was a highly influential example of this effort. Preceding the report, medical education was largely an informal, unregulated "apprenticeship" experience based in a relatively larger number of small schools of varying quality. The Flexner report emphasized specific themes or innovations in medical education, including (1) the mobilization against proprietary medical schools, (2) the importance of the relationship between universities and professional schools, (3) the creation of higher standards for medical school admissions and for highly qualified, full-time faculty, and (4) the movement toward education grounded in scientific research and thinking (Flexner 1910). To this day, the Flexner report still shapes medical as well as dental school curricula.

Increased attention was given to behavioral education in U.S. medical schools as soon as it was recognized that medical care without this element would be inherently less successful (Miller 1955). Despite this realization, the strongly biomedical, scientific educational focus that has been typical in the training and professional socialization of physicians has remained relatively unchanged (Gochman 1997). There is growing recognition of the value of providing a behavioral emphasis in medical and dental education. This change is being incorporated into ongoing reforms of medical curricula in both Europe and the United States (Piko and Kopp 2004).

In dentistry

In Europe, where modern dentistry began, the dentists were primarily trained by apprenticeship, learning by watching and assisting an established dentist. Although self-educated, Pierre Fauchard (1678–1761) exerted a powerful influence to move dentistry forward. During the early 1800s, dental leaders became convinced that dentistry required an enhanced knowledge of science. They further believed that the apprentice method of training was no longer adequate because no one person was both competent to teach all scientific subjects and instruct students in the mechanical techniques of dentistry. This growing understanding subsequently led to the establishment of dental education programs (Fales 2007).

In the United States, 16 years after the aforementioned Flexner report on medical education, the tenth Carnegie report on professional education focused on dentistry (Gies 1926). The Gies report, like the Flexner report, also supported a strong basic science education and almost certainly encouraged dental schools to strengthen this aspect of their curricula. Gies maintained that medicine and dentistry had a common biomedical bond and should be closely aligned. However, he also expressed that the two professions should remain separate since the cultures of physicians and dentists were already well established in the United States and Canada with little interest on the part of either profession to integrate. He further argued that service to the public could best be achieved through a separately organized dental profession; one that he cautioned needed to reform itself in order to elevate dentistry into a respected position in society equal to medicine. Gies also concluded that pre-doctoral education should emphasize general practice and primary care, a focus that still remains strong today.

The development and integration of behaviorally based dental care within the clinical education of students has not been substantial since the middle of the twentieth century.

In the United States, by the middle of the twentieth century, dental caries and periodontal diseases were widespread, with high percentages of patients experiencing rampant caries, abscesses, and advanced periodontitis, all of which created a high rate of edentulism. Because physical removal of caries and tooth extraction were the treatments available, the primary foci of the dental school curriculum were teaching students the skills to extract teeth, physically remove decay, replace the excavated tooth structure with various materials, and create prosthetic devices to replace missing teeth. In the past 60 years, however, the benefits of fluorides have substantially reduced tooth loss and the incidence of caries in all age groups.

Subsequently, more recent observations of curricular practices and needs in dentistry were reviewed (Tedesco 1995) as groundwork for the historic Institute of Medicine report on the future of dental education (Field 1995). Since the 1930s, behavioral sciences have been included among the essential elements in dental education. Yet the growth, development, and integration of behaviorally based dental care within the clinical education of students has not been substantial since that time. Lack of focus and time spent on health behavior does not result from a lack of guidelines. Professional associations and some dental schools have issued guidelines over the past 2 decades. These guidelines provide competency expectations and curricular goals for a wide range of topics, including the dynamics of dentist-patient interactions and the characteristics of patient behaviors (Plasschaert et al. 2005; Tedesco 1995).

In dental hygiene

It was recognized early that providing individual preventive care in dentistry could be time consuming. In 1911, Alfred C. Fones was the first dentist to formalize a role for auxiliary dental personnel in educating and instructing their patients. Fones also developed the first formal educational program for dental hygienists in 1913. Prevention, patient education, and behavioral guidance have always been central and defining roles for dental hygienists. In the United States, many of the early community health education programs that utilized dental hygienists focused on children in schools. The literature provides little information about the specific activities of early dental hygienists in private practice (Fales 2007).

HEALTH BEHAVIOR CHANGE EDUCATION

Today, the roles of dental hygienists are many and varied (Mueller-Joseph et al. 2005), but in brief, among them are

- educator/health promoter: use educational theory and methods to analyze health needs, develop health promotion strategies, and deliver and evaluate the results of attaining or maintaining oral health for individuals or groups; and

- change agent: analyze barriers to change, develop mechanisms to effect change, implement processes and evaluate successes of programs that promote health for individuals, families, or communities, and promote lifestyle for individual changes.

Although the strength and importance of creating and maintaining a productive professional alliance between dentists and dental hygienists may seem obvious, it was not until 1992 that behavioral objectives for dental education were developed recommending that dental students be taught to "consult with and refer to dental hygienists those patients needing nonsurgical periodontal therapy and supportive periodontal treatment" (Fales 2007).

CURRENTS TRENDS IN DENTAL CARE AND EDUCATION

During the last 30–40 years, there has been a substantial improvement in oral cleanliness in many countries. For some, oral hygiene "exercises" are as much part of routine health behaviors as weight control, exercise, smoking cessation, and other modification of lifestyle. All of these interventions are aimed at an improved quality of life, a healthier body, and increased lifespan. In Europe, behavioral medicine has traditionally been most strongly emphasized in the Netherlands and the Scandinavian countries (Piko and Kopp 2004), with considerable differences in the oral hygiene emphasis between and within countries, mainly explained by traditions, cultural traits, and social ambience (Löe 2000).

There is a great diversity in the methods, standards, and outcomes of dental education systems throughout the world. The "straight from secondary school to dental school" model, so common in parts of Europe and the ex-colonies, is very different from the post-baccalaureate system of dental education (Reed et al. 2002). The "odontological" approach to dental education, with little or no attachment to medicine, has historically been most prevalent in the

Americas, much of Africa, the Western Pacific, certain Asian countries, and some European countries, particularly those in the north and west. Conversely, the "stomatological" approach to dental education, which incorporates dentistry into medical education in a way similar to that of other specialty medical subjects, has been prevalent elsewhere, including the countries of eastern and central Europe.

With the development of the European Union (EU), the directives of the European Commission (EC) required dental education in some areas (for example, Austria, Spain, Portugal, and Italy) to change from a stomatological educational model to an independent, odontological educational process. Paradoxically, however, while some dental curricula taught in the stomatological model have reduced the scope of the medical instruction in their schools, many traditionally odontological dental schools have been striving to bolster the "medical" elements of their programs. Little objective evidence exists regarding the extent to which the use of the stomatological or odontological approach to dental education may be beneficial or otherwise in reducing oral health disparities or increasing access to care (Hobdell et al. 2002).

Voluntary efforts among European dental schools to perform self-assessments ultimately aimed at creating common educational standards for European dental education (the DentEd thematic network project) revealed persistent educational disparities (Shanley and Nattestad 2002). Postgraduate vocational training programs for new graduates under the supervision of established clinicians to assist in the transition from the relatively sheltered environment of dental school to the pressures of independent practice have been required in some EU countries (Scott 2003).

In the United States today, the traditional external outcome measures reflecting the success of training in dentistry have been both state and national dental board exams. Often curricular emphasis has been justified in terms of the content included in these licensing examinations. Unfortunately, however, these exams include little focus on evaluating behavioral aspects in patient care, thus, this educational focus remains under-represented in many dental schools' curricula (Gift and White 1997).

Traditional technological approaches to dental education must give greater expression to the psychosocial imperatives of health care while adapting to new and rapidly emerging research findings (Shanley and Nattestad 2002) and reflecting cultural, demographic, financial, and environmental circumstances of each individual school and country (Manogue et al. 2002).

HEALTH BEHAVIOR CHANGE
EDUCATION

THE NEED FOR CHANGE IN DENTAL EDUCATION

Public health goals and responsibilities

Traditionally, the goal of health care interventions has been to "cure" the patient. However, since chronic and behaviorally based diseases have become so prominent in modern society, this narrow criterion of success is no longer sufficient. As outlined in chapter 1, cure is neither essential nor necessary in order that the patient may benefit from health care interventions. Training of dental professionals has also traditionally been focused on clinician-rendered treatment for disease rather than assisting people to change their behavior. Assisting patients in developing and practicing favorable health behaviors may constitute the more meaningful role in many aspects of health care (Mann and Stuenkel 2006).

Patient self-management strategies and interactive methods to encourage informed patient choice are rapidly developing areas in health care. In order for such changes to be implemented in dental practice, changes in both the professional training and cultural norms in dental care will be needed.

    Patient self-management strategies and interactive methods to encourage evidence-based informed patient choice, on the other hand, are rapidly developing areas in health care that may hold both economic and philosophical advantages (Redman 2007). In order for such changes to be implemented, changes in both the professional training and cultural norms in health care will still be needed.

New educational initiatives and methods

Organizing a curriculum that emphasizes and fosters students' capacities to perform optimally and independently may be based on either a "bottom-up" or a "top-down" educational structure (Hendricson and Cohen 2001). In the traditional "bottom-up" instructional process, the teaching is organized into topic-specific "silos" (traditional courses). The content of each course is determined primarily by the course director, an expert in that particular area of study, in response to the question, "What do I want to teach students about my chosen field?" In contrast, in the "top-down" curricular approach, the educational content is determined based on a formal analysis of the health care

To provide an educational environment that will allow students to independently provide behavior change strategies in the practice of dentistry, a specific curriculum must be created and implemented to encourage such strategies.

needs of the local society and the responsibilities and tasks of working health care professionals.

The content is then driven by the specific knowledge, skills, and values required to perform these professional measures. Focused learning activities are then designed to provide students with the experiences to attain and demonstrate competency. With this, the education is designed in answer to the questions, "What must graduates be able to do so they can function as entry-level clinicians without direct supervision or coaching?" or "What must our graduates be able to do so they can provide patient care and benefit from educational experiences at the next level of professional training?" (Hendricson and Cohen 2001).

In order to provide an educational environment that will allow students to independently provide behavior change strategies in the practice of dentistry, a specific curriculum must be created and implemented to encourage such strategies. In general, a knowledge base providing a background of theoretical education must be attained. Along with this, clinical instruction must be provided and clinical practice assessed. As an example, the application of such strategies specifically to the teaching of tobacco use cessation has been elaborated on at the First European Workshop on Tobacco Use Prevention and Cessation for Oral Health Professionals (Ramseier et al. 2006a, 2006b).

THEORETICAL EDUCATION

Pathology and epidemiology of diseases

In general, for health behavior change curricula, a knowledge base attained through lectures, Problem-Based Learning (PBL), or E-Learning and clinical skills attained through clinical instructions and practices are required.

All dental education programs provide significant biomedical background for students on specific etiologies, pathological mechanisms, and morbid outcomes of common oral diseases. The study of epidemiology detailing the concentration of disease risk factors within certain groups or linked to certain behaviors is a further standard component of all dental curricula. Despite the fact that dental students are well versed in these basic concepts related to the disease risk, causation, and distribution, their ability to translate and apply them appropriately and effectively during patient care has not been commonly emphasized nor routinely assessed. Thus, teaching goals and strategies within suggested educational settings and formats may be valuable. The further development and assessment of both knowledge and skills may assist in the understanding and effective management of oral diseases.

Behavior as a determinant of health and disease

It is generally recognized that the success of health care, in part, depends on the patient's willingness to acknowledge responsibility to carry out recommended behaviors. Many factors must be considered in the formulation of these behavioral strategies. One factor is the increased cost of care if patients are non-compliant. While health behavior research has improved the understanding of dentist-patient interactions and other critical issues surrounding provision of care, more often than not, the research findings have not been applied in professional education, training, or practice (Gift and White 1997).

Illness may affect all aspects of an individual's life. However, the impact felt by each individual may differ due to personality traits, beliefs and values, the available support system, and other factors unique to the individual. "Illness behavior" is influenced by a patient's health beliefs. In the "impaired role," patients must take responsibility for their own health and can meet normal role expectations within the limits of their condition in the form of "adapted wellness" (Larsen et al. 2006).

A prominent hypothesis in the study of social inequalities in health is that elevated risk among the socio-economically disadvantaged is largely the result of the higher prevalence of health risk behaviors (and the lack of health-promoting behaviors) among those with lower levels of income (Hobdell et al. 2002). Inequalities in oral health are marked among adults, with people from disadvantaged backgrounds being significantly more likely to have more untreated dental caries, fewer fillings, and more missing teeth (Brown 1994).

Health professionals' attitudes are representative of general societal views and so can be expected to include prejudices (Mann and Stuenkel 2006). Health professional students' perspectives have shown a surprisingly high level of *stigma* associated with illness. Studies of students have revealed concerns over the perception of social stigma attached to their own personal health and the resulting professional jeopardy that they may encounter upon disclosure. This perception suggests that, when the health professional feels that he or she has a lot to risk, the fear of being stigmatized is greater and the resistance to de-stigmatizing efforts may be greater (Mann & Stuenkel 2006).

Research has confirmed that the relationship between socio-economic inequalities and health is partly mediated by lifestyle factors closely connected to psychological factors such as hopelessness and depression. Recently a focus of behavioral epidemiological research has turned to protective factors, namely social support, spirituality, and social capital. These protective factors have a strong influence on health risk behaviors, psychosomatic symptoms, self-rated health, and mortality (Piko and Kopp 2004).

PRACTICAL EDUCATION

Dental educators tend to be empiricists (i.e., their own personal experience strongly influences their decisions to accept new information or adopt innovation). This fact affects not only clinical patient care decisions but also decisions regarding instructional philosophies and methods. Such an empirical approach may tend to slow adaptation to and adoption of change. These observed trends are only natural for current faculty members because they are largely the products of an empirical clinical educational approach during their own training (Bader and Shugars 1995).

A survey conducted by the American Dental Education Association (ADEA) regarding tobacco prevention and cessation in U.S. dental schools was reported by Weaver, Whittaker, Valachovic, and Broom in 2002 (Weaver et al. 2002). The authors described the barriers to the schools' efforts in preparing students to intervene in their patients' tobacco use. The survey revealed that a general lack of faculty preparation hindered this process. Considering the fundamental role of dental educators in teaching their students about tobacco use prevention and cessation skills, the need for faculty preparation appears to be evident.

Students

Dental education has been focusing on technical competence rather than problem solving and interaction skills (Tedesco 1995). Students possessing technical skills fit in well with the prevailing educational process in dental schools but may not be well suited for the development of adequate communication and related interpersonal skills. A critical step between the classroom and the clinical setting is the application and integration of didactic principles in patient care and communication (Gift and White 1997).

HEALTH BEHAVIOR CHANGE EDUCATION

Observational experiences are an important mechanism of influencing health care students' behaviors. Students' assessments of their own abilities will depend on the talents of those they choose to observe and to model and with whom they make comparisons. When students compare themselves to clinical mentors, they tend to identify with these mentors. Seeing a mentor perform successfully will inspire confidence among students that they may also have the capabilities to perform equally well (Bandura 1997).

The first implementation of a tobacco cessation program developed by the U.S. National Cancer Institute was in 1993, as reported and evaluated by Barker, Taylor, and Barker in 1995 (Barker et al. 1995). The program objectives were (1) to encourage dental students to ask patients about tobacco habits, (2) advise patients against tobacco use, and (3) assist interested patients in the tobacco cessation process. Both faculty and students were actively involved in the implementation process, with follow-up lectures and feedback sessions to discuss perceived barriers at regular intervals. The authors concluded that this implementation process was successful and may also be applicable to other dental schools.

Health behavior change program in the student clinics

Recently at the University of Michigan School of Dentistry, a new program has been designed, developed, and implemented to encourage faculty and students to adopt a method and foster a culture to support, practice, and formally evaluate health behavior change strategies in the routine care of patients in the student clinics. The entire process is intended to assess the students' skills to plan and conduct a patient-centered interview and implement behavioral change strategies for patients to reduce oral health–related behavioral risk factors.

The health behavior change program is an adaptation of the model described by Ramseier and co-workers (Ramseier et al. 2006a) for tobacco cessation and utilizes aspects of

• the model "stages of change" (or transtheoretical model) introduced by Prochaska and DiClemente in 1983 (Prochaska and DiClemente 1983);

• the five As (Ask, Advise, Assess, Assist, and Arrange) described in the clinical practice guideline by Fiore and co-authors (Fiore 2000); and

• the main principles of Motivational Interviewing techniques described by Miller and Rollnick in 1991 and 2002 (Miller and Rollnick 2002).

Patients in active periodontal treatment and/or currently using tobacco products are eligible for involvement in the health behavior change program. Before the formal behavioral intervention commences, students prepare a brief written outline describing the intended goals and the process by which these goals may be achieved as well as anticipated talking points. The instructor reviews this outline and then observes and critiques the student's one-on-one health behavior change interview.

Given the nature of time constraints in the dental teaching clinics, the health behavior change interview is planned to last more than 5 but less than 15 minutes. The instructor does not participate in the discussion in any way but will seek to observe the following features of the interaction:

- Motivation: the student engages the patient in an interview about health behavior change. When approaching the patient with questions targeting certain health behaviors, the student elicits indicators of the patient's motivation to change.

- Confidence: with patients willing to change, the student continues to ask about the patients' confidence to successfully change. Less confident patients will be asked about their personal advantages if they were to change. More confident patients will receive further counselling according to their needs, such as specific plaque and/or diet information or a tobacco use cessation protocol for those who are using tobacco.

- Permission: with patients unwilling or less confident to change, the student asks about permission to ask about health behavior change again at a following visit.

In the Michigan model for health behavior change student assessment, the tobacco use cessation protocol also aims to adapt the Assist and the Arrange of the 5 As. In brief, it consists of

- asking the patient to fill in a smoking control journal,

- evaluating the smoking control journal at any following visit,

- discussing targeted behavioral changes and the use of nicotine replacement therapy at any following visit, and

- confirming or redefining the nicotine replacement measures found and scheduling the quit date at any following visit.

Following the observations of the health behavior change interview, faculty members critique the student's efforts using a standardized form (Figure 7.1 and Table 7.1). Specific feedback is provided in each of the following categories:

- patient engagement,

- risk assessment,

- appropriate patient information,

- personalized self-care instruction, and

- clinical protocol and professionalism.

Clinical faculty training

Background information and the prescribed protocols for this educational process were initially presented to the attending clinical faculty members as a group. Following this, students were also provided with a formal introduction to the health behavior change interviewing process and the associated exercises in a classroom setting.

Despite some initial misgivings expressed by a few faculty members regarding a lack of confidence in participating in a "new" process based on their prior background and training, initial impressions regarding this educational initiative suggest that cultural changes related to this program may yield enhanced sensitivity and attentiveness to the health behavior change process at the institutional level and hopefully beyond.

CONTINUING EDUCATION

Clinicians

Repetitive assessment of values, attitudes, and skills is a part of training for all health care professionals. The professional opinions and behaviors of oral health care providers are modelled by their individual backgrounds, ethics, and beliefs. As patients, they have generally expected and likely observed high standards of conduct from their own professional colleagues. Because a variety of forces establish and later influence normative patterns of practice behavior

Health Behavior Change Performance Exam

Student: _____ Clinic_____ Date_____
Pt. Name:_____ Chart #:_____ ADA Proc. Code_____
Instructor Name (printed) _____
Instructor Signature_____

Enter grades and optional comments in the boxes to the right of each question:

Professionalism Ratings	Grading Criteria		Comments (Required for V)	GRADE
Preparedness	R	Ready for patient care		
	S	1 error		
	V	2 or more errors		
Patient Management	R	Follows HIPAA protocol		
	S	Minor errors		
	V	Patient care compromised		
Infection Control	R	Follows OSHA guidelines		
	S	Minor errors		
	V	Patient care compromised		

Specific Questions	Grading Criteria		Comments (Required for V)	GRADE
Current Oral Health Status	R	Status explained clearly		
	S	Status explained superficially		
	V	Status not discussed		
Habits, History, and Rationale	R	Thorough history, explanation		
	S	Cursory history, explanation		
	V	No history, explanation		
Motivation and Confidence	R	Thoroughly investigated		
	S	Superficially investigated		
	V	Not investigated		
Goals, Process, and Follow-Up Plan	R	Clear goals, process, plans		
	S	Vague goals, process, plans		
	V	No goals, process, plans		
Interactive Style and Professionalism	R	Good interaction, rapport		
	S	Dominance or detachment		
	V	Unilateral or inappropriate		

Figure 7.1. Health behavior change performance exam evaluation sheet.

Table 7.1. Health behavior change performance exam evaluation criteria table.

	Criteria for Health Behavior Change		
	R (It's All Good)	S (Minor Concerns)	V (Major Errors)
Current Oral Health Status	The patient has a current oral health concern related to behavior (periodontally unstable, caries unstable, or using tobacco products)	The patient has a current oral health concern related to behavior (periodontally unstable, caries unstable, or using tobacco products)	The patient does not have an oral health concern related to behavior or the patient's current health status was not discussed with him or her
	The patient's current health status is clearly explained to him or her	The patient's current health status is explained to him or but only superficially	
Habits, History, and Rationale	The student thoroughly investigates and documents the patient's behavioral history (plaque control habits, dietary habits, tobacco habits), past therapeutic interventions, and associated lifestyle and other issues	The student only briefly investigates the patient's behavioral history (plaque control habits, dietary habits, tobacco habits), past therapeutic interventions, and associated lifestyle and other issues	The student fails to gather or document any meaningful history or lifestyle information
	The patient is provided with a complete explanation of how specific behavioral factors contribute to disease	The patient is provided with a superficial explanation of how specific behavioral factors contribute to disease	The patient is provided with no explanation of how behavior may influence disease

Motivation and Confidence	The patient is specifically engaged and asked to share his or her motivation for behavioral change Less confident patients are asked to consider potential advantages of behavioral change More confident patients are given further behavioral change counselling according to their specific needs	Patient motivation and confidence are explored but only superficially Patient consideration or professional counselling are pursued appropriately based on what was learned	Patient motivation and confidence are not explored A unidirectional behavioral change counselling effort is actively pursued by the student, despite a potential lack of patient motivation and/or confidence
Goals, Process, and Follow-Up Plan	Specific behavioral change goals are established including significant patient input Specific health behavior changes are clearly specified/demonstrated, appropriate for the needs, motivation, and confidence of the patient A specific follow-up plan is established to revisit, monitor, or maintain behavioral practices	Non-specific behavioral change goals are discussed with limited patient involvement Health behavior changes are suggested, appropriate for the needs, motivation, and confidence of the patient, but clarity and/or technique could be improved Follow-up plans regarding health behavior practices are discussed, but only non-specifically	No mutually agreed-upon goals are established following the intervention No health behavior changes are specified/demonstrated or clarity and/or technique is inappropriate for the needs, motivation, and/or confidence of the patient No plans for health behavior follow-up are made
Clinical Protocol and Professionalism	Productive interaction between student and patient The student demonstrates sincerity and attentiveness regarding the patient's condition and needs The student establishes good rapport with the patient	The student or the patient is overly dominant in the interaction and planning process The student appears slightly detached The interaction seems slightly superficial	The patient does not participate in the interaction The student demonstrates inappropriate clinical behavior The student is deceptive or behaves in a clearly unprofessional manner

in health care, researchers have been unable to formulate a unifying theory of clinician behavior change, applicable and successfully proven among practicing professionals (Smith 2000).

There is limited understanding of the ways in which dental professionals obtain new information about behaviors and the barriers to the incorporation of this knowledge into clinical practice. Until ways are found to translate research findings into action, few changes in behavioral skills will be seen in the dental profession. Continuing education programs that could help address gaps in professional behavioral skills training have met with varying degrees of success. Often those dentists who may be most in need of training do not select the courses that address communication and behavior management skills. Enhancing dentists' skills in acknowledging, interpreting, and acting on patient information and motivations, as well as more behavioral research in the education of oral health professionals throughout the career cycle, is still needed (Gift and White 1997).

Motivating the practicing dental team to get involved in tobacco use cessation involves three key elements referred to as the 3 Ts (Wickholm et al. 2006). These elements are:

- Tension: creating a motivational tension so that the dental team wants to get involved.

- Triggers: populating the environment of the dental team with reminders and prompts that translate the motivation into action.

- Training: ensuring that the dental team has the confidence, skills, and knowledge to do it effectively.

Practical demonstration of how the dental health team can be motivated to receive training in tobacco cessation within these three themes and evidence of the effectiveness of these methods has been described (Wickholm et al. 2006). These authors propose and describe two different levels of tobacco use cessation instruction that may be provided in continuing education programs:

- Brief advice training: asking patients about their tobacco use, advising them to stop, and assisting them or referring them to specialist tobacco use cessation services if available.

- Enhanced interventions: incorporating the elements of brief advice, possibly including more intensive assistance, as well as including attempts to motivate patients using tobacco to make a quit attempt.

Although clear evidence of widespread success for these or other strategies aimed at expanding the capacities, participation, and success of dental health professionals in tobacco use cessation may still be lacking, this fact should not preclude their use.

ASSESSMENT OF HEALTH BEHAVIOR CHANGE EDUCATION

Faculty

The relationship between a student's competence and an instructor's competence is entangled in the evaluation process. To some extent this relationship depends upon who is regarded as more responsible for the learning (Redman 2007). An equally potent force is the "hidden curriculum," described as the unintended and sometimes negative consequences of the structure of the educational process, particularly the methods of assessment and teaching as well as the attitudes of the teachers (Manogue et al. 2002).

> Assessment universally drives the process of learning. Whatever the circumstances, all educators must focus on what graduates need for optimum performance and lifelong self-development through active learning while being accountable to the society they must serve as ethical clinicians.

Assessment universally drives the process of learning. Whatever the circumstances, all educators must focus on what graduates need for optimum performance and lifelong self-development through active learning while being accountable to the society they must serve as ethical clinicians (Shanley and Nattestad 2002). A major factor in enabling continuous quality improvement in education is the availability of information on best practices and access to the evidence for their acceptability (Manogue et al. 2002).

Students

In undergraduate and graduate education of dentists and dental hygienists, assessment should target both the knowledge base and the necessary skills for behavioral change counselling and communication. Such an assessment should be placed as early in the curriculum as possible to emphasize the importance of these interventions as part of clinical practice (Ramseier et al. 2006a). There is an absence of literature in dentistry as to why particular methods of assessment are used. Simply changing the method of assessment may cause tensions when traditional instructional methods remain unchanged (Manogue et al. 2002).

One approach to skills assessment for behavior change education is the concept proposed by Miller in his "competence pyramid" (Miller 1990). At the base of the pyramid is background knowledge that can be assessed with summative or factual tests. The next step up the pyramid is to assess the capacity to understand and perform component tasks of the intervention that may take place in a pre-clinical or simulation environment. Both these categories of performance are representative of the cognitive domain of learning. Beyond this, the remaining steps up the pyramid enter the behavioral domain of skill development and assessment. First, the ability to integrate and effectively perform the behavior change intervention must be assessed in a clinical setting. Finally, the independent utilization of behavior change methods in routine clinical practice may also be evaluated with case presentations in the patient care environment. As learners progress through the ascending stages of the pyramid, they derive increasing professional authenticity with every successive step.

Clinicians

Researchers have found evidence that health care providers contemplating and/or adopting behavior change attend continuing education courses primarily to validate and test the reliability of their learning and behavior, either that of new information and innovations or that of what they are already doing in practice. However, such passive educational strategies have not been found to be effective. Education in small doses is likely ineffective because it cannot compete with the extensive body of background and experience driving professional behavior that clinicians already possess (Smith 2000).

Evidence-based guidelines are intended to change behavior by providing definitive information on best practices from authoritative sources to well-trained, interested, logical clinicians. Research has shown that simple provision of information in the form of guidelines is also insufficient to affect individual behavior patterns. Such educational strategies may be most appropriate for early stage adopters, whereas enabling strategies such as reminders may be most appropriate for late-stage adopters. Additionally, literature reviews have suggested that reminders (paper, electronic) provided to health care professionals may demonstrate the best evidence of consistent effectiveness of clinician behavior change (Smith 2000).

There is good evidence from systematic reviews of the effectiveness of smoking cessation training programs being multi-component and including elements of outreach (training in the health professional's practice) and combining educational and practice-based learning (Anderson and Jane-Llopis 2004). The provision of prompts and reminders following training appears to enhance the effectiveness of such training (Lancaster et al. 2000). There is also some evidence that prompts can be effective in increasing the rate of brief tobacco use advice provided by primary health care professionals (McEwen et al. 2002).

SUMMARY

The primary foci of the dental school curricula in the middle of the twentieth century were teaching students the skills to extract teeth, physically remove decay, replace the excavated tooth structure with various materials, and create prosthetic devices to replace missing teeth. Today, patient self-management strategies and interactive methods to encourage informed patient choice are rapidly developing areas in health care. In order for such changes to be implemented in dental practice, changes in both the professional training and cultural norms in dental care are needed. In general, for health behavior change curricula, a knowledge base attained through lectures, Problem-Based Learning, or E-Learning and clinical skills attained through clinical instructions and practices are required. Concerning the assessment of dental and dental hygiene students, all educators must focus on what graduates need for optimum performance and lifelong self-development through active learning while being accountable to the society they must serve as ethical clinicians.

REFERENCES

Anderson, P., and E. Jane-Llopis. (2004). How can we increase the involvement of primary health care in the treatment of tobacco dependence? A meta-analysis. *Addiction* 99(3):299–312.

Bader, J.D., and D.A. Shugars. (1995). Variation, treatment outcomes, and practice guidelines in dental practice. *J Dent Educ* 59(1):61–95.

Bandura, A. (1997). *Self-Efficacy: The Exercise of Control.* New York: W.H. Freeman.

Barker, G.J., T.S. Taylor, et al. (1995). Implementation of a tobacco cessation program in the student clinics. *J Dent Educ* 59(8):850–855.

Brown, L.F. (1994). Research in dental health education and health promotion: A review of the literature. *Health Educ Q* 21(1):83–102.

Fales, M.H. (2007). Historical perspectives on dental hygiene and periodontology. In: D.A. Perry and P.L. Beemsterboer, *Periodontology for the Dental Hygienist*. St. Louis: Saunders Elsevier, 3–23.

Field, M.J. (ed.). (1995). *Dental Education at the CrossroadsemChallenges and Change*. Washington, DC: National Academy Press.

Fiore, M.C. (2000). US public health service clinical practice guideline: Treating tobacco use and dependence. *Respir Care* 45(10):1200–1262.

Flexner, A. (ed.). (1910). *Medical Education in the United States and Canada: A Report to the Carnegie Foundation for the Advancement of Teaching*. Boston: Merrymount Press.

Gies, W.J. (ed.). (1926). *Dental Education in the U.S. and Canada: A Report to the Carnegie Foundation for the Advancement of Teaching*. New York: Carnegie Foundation for the Advancement of Teaching.

Gift, H.C., and B.A. White. (1997). Health behavior research and oral health. In: D.S. Gochman, *Handbook of Health Behavior Research, IV: Relevance for Professionals and Issues for the Future*. New York: Plenum Press, 121–142.

Gochman, D.S. (1997). *Professional training and practice*. New York: Plenum Press.

Gochman, D.S. (1997). Relevance of health behavior research. *Handbook of Health Behavior Research, IV: Relevance for Professionals and Issues for the Future*. New York: Plenum Press, 377–393.

Hendricson, W.D., and P.A. Cohen. (2001). Oral health care in the 21st century: Implications for dental and medical education. *Acad Med* 76(12):1181–1206.

Hobdell, M., J. Sinkford, et al. (2002). 5.2 Ethics, equity and global responsibilities in oral health and disease. *Eur J Dent Educ* 6 Suppl 3:167–178.

Lancaster, T., C. Silagy, et al. (2000). Training health professionals in smoking cessation. *Cochrane Database Syst Rev*(3), CD000214.

Larsen, P.D., P.R. Lewis, et al. (2006). Illness behavior and roles. In: I.M. Lubkin and P.D. Larsen, *Chronic Illness: Impact and Interventions*. Sudbury, MA: Jones and Bartlett, 23–44.

Löe, H. (2000). Oral hygiene in the prevention of caries and periodontal disease. *Int Dent J* 50(3):129–139.

Mann, R.J., and D. Stuenkel. (2006). Stigma. In: I.M. Lubkin and P.D. Larsen, *Chronic Illness: Impact and Interventions*. Sudbury, MA: Jones and Bartlett, 45–66.

Manogue, M., M. Kelly, et al. (2002). 2.1 Evolving methods of assessment. *Eur J Dent Educ* 6 Suppl 3:53–66.

McEwen, A., A. Preston, et al. (2002). Effect of a GP desktop resource on smoking cessation activities of general practitioners. *Addiction* 97(5):595–597.

Miller, G.E. (1990). The assessment of clinical skills/competence/performance. *Acad Med*(Supplement 9):63–67.

Miller, J.G. (1955). Toward a general theory for the behavioral sciences. *Am Psychol* 10:513–531.

Miller, W.R., and S. Rollnick (eds.). (2002). *Motivational Interviewing: Preparing People for Change*, 2nd ed. New York: Guilford Press.

Mueller-Joseph, L., D.F. Homenko, et al. (2005). The professional dental hygienist. *Clinical Practice of the Dental Hygienist*. Philadelphia: Lippincott Williams & Wilkins, 3–14.

Piko, B.F., and M.S. Kopp. (2004). Paradigm shifts in medical and dental education: Behavioural sciences and behavioural medicine. *Eur J Dent Educ* 8 Suppl 4:25–31.

Plasschaert, A.J., W.P. Holbrook, et al. (2005). Profile and competences for the European dentist. *Eur J Dent Educ* 9(3):98–107.

Prochaska, J.O., and C.C. DiClemente. (1983). Stages and processes of self-change of smoking: Toward an integrative model of change. *J Consult Clin Psychol* 51(3):390–395.

Ramseier, C.A., A. Christen, et al. (2006a). Tobacco use prevention and cessation in dental and dental hygiene undergraduate education. *Oral Health Prev Dent* 4(1):49–60.

Ramseier, C.A., N. Mattheos, et al. (2006b). Consensus report: First European Workshop on Tobacco Use Prevention and Cessation for Oral Health Professionals. *Oral Health Prev Dent* 4(1):7–18.

Redman, B. K. (2007). *The Practice of Patient Education: A Case Study Approach.* St. Louis: Mosby.

Reed, M., N. Claffey, et al. (2002). 2.3 Towards global convergence of education, training, quality, outcome and assessment. *Eur J Dent Educ* 6 Suppl 3:78–83.

Scott, J. (2003). Dental education in Europe: The challenges of variety. *J Dent Educ* 67(1):69–78.

Shanley, D., and A. Nattestad. (2002). Introduction: A global congress in dental education. *Eur J Dent Educ* 6 Suppl 3:5–6.

Smith, W.R. (2000). Evidence for the effectiveness of techniques to change physician behavior. *Chest* 118(2 Suppl):8S–17S.

Tedesco, L.A. (1995). Issues in dental curriculum development and change. *J Dent Educ* 59(1):97–147.

Weaver, R.G., L. Whittaker, et al. (2002). Tobacco control and prevention effort in dental education. *J Dent Educ* 66(3):426–429.

Wickholm, S., A. McEwen, et al. (2006). Continuing education of tobacco use cessation (TUC) for dentists and dental hygienists. *Oral Health Prev Dent* 4(1):61–70.

HEALTH BEHAVIOR CHANGE EDUCATION

INDEX

Printed in the United States
By Bookmasters

Printed in the United States
By Bookmasters